How the Other Half Eats

THE UNTOLD STORY OF FOOD AND INEQUALITY IN AMERICA

"*How the Other Half Eats* is a must-read for anyone who has ever wondered why Americans don't eat more healthfully. Fielding-Singh achieved something remarkable in gaining the trust of families who then let her observe their daily food choices. Her book is a thoughtful, riveting, compassionate, and utterly compelling account of why eating healthfully is so difficult, especially for the poor. What's more, she offers a superb example of why on-the-ground field research is invaluable for gaining a deep and nuanced understanding of the ways that our industry-driven and highly inequitable food environment affects real people on a daily basis."

—Marion Nestle, author of *Let's Ask Marion*

"Deeply empathetic…a devastating portrait of 'the scarcity, uncertainty, and anxiety that permeate so much of the American dietary experience.'" —*Publishers Weekly* (starred review)

"Bold, eye-opening, and deeply moving, *How the Other Half Eats* is a must-read for anyone concerned about the well-being of American families. Fielding-Singh powerfully shows how sweeping, systemic inequities find their way onto our dinner plates and affect our health and wellness. This compassionate and captivating book resonated with me as a physician caring for my patients and as a mother striving to do right by my children."

—Leana Wen, MD, author of *Lifelines*

"Illuminating." —Jessica Grose, *New York Times*

"Fielding-Singh draws on years of meticulous field research, statistics, and her own experience as a mother and biracial South Asian American woman to detail the constraints and challenges all mothers face in providing healthy, nourishing, and enjoyable meals for their children and families... She dispels the myth that access to good food is the primary driver of the nation's food and health disparities... *How the Other Half Eats* weaves lyrical storytelling and fascinating research into a compelling narrative that shows the devastating impact—physical, emotional, and economic—our industrial food system has not just on the 'other half,' but upon us all."

—Beth Dooley, *San Francisco Chronicle*

"If you think that poor health, obesity, and bad food choices are a matter of personal responsibility, *How the Other Half Eats* will make you think again. Through the stories of four families struggling to feed themselves, Fielding-Singh vividly brings to light the human aspect of our disordered food system and the structural challenges of poverty and lack of education about access to real food in this examination of the fundamental flaws in our food system. We live in a country where we throw out one-third of our food, yet one in four children are food-insecure. The complex web of social, political, and economic conditions that give rise to massive nutrition and food insecurity comes to life in this book. It should be mandatory reading for parents, teachers, health-care workers, and policymakers."

—Mark Hyman, MD, author of *The Pegan Diet*

"Reveals the thin tightrope that parents—mostly mothers—must walk to feed their children while maintaining their dignity and sense of worth, even as others judge and critique their food choices." —*Food52*

"An eye-opening and intimate study of what families eat and why." — *Kirkus Reviews*

"*How the Other Half Eats* overturns the conventional wisdom about childhood obesity, food deserts, and nutritional inequality, replacing it with a profound and compelling ground truth. Fielding-Singh shows us how inequalities in families' diets do not stem from the negligence of some parents and the devotion of others. Rather, the food that graces the plates of all children—rich and poor, Black and white—reflects mothers' deep-seated love and commitment to their kids' well-being. Honest, incisive, and illuminating, *How the Other Half Eats* is the book we need about food and inequality in America."
—Kathryn Edin, author of *$2.00 a Day*

"In this intimate and revealing chronicle, Fielding-Singh has done us a great service by revealing myth-busting truths about poverty, wealth, hunger, and abundance. More than that, she does it in a way that shows how knowledge might be shared compassionately, in the best tradition of engaged scholar activism. This isn't just undercover journalism, but an epistemology of the American dining table. After reading it, you'll never be able to claim you didn't know, or know how to know, how the other half eats." —Raj Patel, author of *Stuffed and Starved*

How the Other Half Eats

THE UNTOLD STORY OF FOOD AND INEQUALITY IN AMERICA

PRIYA FIELDING-SINGH, PhD

Little, Brown Spark

New York Boston London

For Josh, who beat the odds

Little, Brown Spark
Hachette Book Group
1290 Avenue of the Americas, New York, NY 10104
littlebrownspark.com

Originally published in hardcover by Little, Brown Spark, November 2021
First Little Brown, Spark paperback edition, May 2023

Little, Brown Spark is an imprint of Little, Brown and Company, a division of Hachette Book Group, Inc. The Little, Brown Spark name and logo are trademarks of Hachette Book Group, Inc.

The publisher is not responsible for websites (or their content) that are not owned by the publisher.

The Hachette Speakers Bureau provides a wide range of authors for speaking events. To find out more, go to hachettespeakersbureau.com or email hachettespeakers@hbgusa.com.

Little, Brown and Company books may be purchased in bulk for business, educational, or promotional use. For information, please contact your local bookseller or the Hachette Book Group Special Markets Department at special.markets@hbgusa.com.

ISBN 9780316427265 (hardcover) / 9780316427258 (paperback)
LCCN 2021938481

Printing 1, 2023

LSC-C

Printed in the United States of America

we are each other's harvest:
we are each other's business:
we are each other's magnitude and bond.

— Gwendolyn Brooks, "Paul Robeson"

What I want is so simple I almost can't say it: elementary kindness. Enough to eat, enough to go around. The possibility that kids might one day grow up to be neither the destroyers nor the destroyed.

— Barbara Kingsolver, *Animal Dreams*

Contents

Preface

Outstretched on a hospital bed, I clutched Veda's slippery body close to my chest as she stared up at me for the first time, her wrinkly right hand wrapped around my thumb. At six pounds, five ounces and twenty-one inches long, my daughter stretched from my collar down to my hip bone. I took her in, admiring her full head of thick black hair, ten scaly fingers, ten stubby toes, and the surfboard-shaped birthmark above her left thigh. As I stared into her soft brown eyes, my heart swelled. *It's you,* I thought. *It's been you all along.*

The moment I met Veda was the moment I discovered a new, surprising kind of love. I had known the love a daughter feels toward her parents, a sister toward her brothers, and a wife toward her husband. But this love felt different. It was searingly visceral and uniquely overwhelming. For months, I had envisioned what feelings might arise upon finally meeting my daughter. I knew that I would care deeply for her. But what made my love for Veda distinct was this: At its core was an enormous, at times overpowering, feeling of responsibility. From her first moments resting on my chest up until today, I have not been able to separate my love for my daughter from the immense ownership I feel for her well-being.

Pregnancy provided the training grounds for this feeling. As Veda grew inside of me over the course of nine months, my sense of responsibility for her also ballooned. My body was her home. We were separate people, but we were inseparable. That inseparability made it challenging for me to act without first considering that action's impact on her. I longed to be a self-assured, composed pregnant woman who "trusted the process" and knew her baby would be fine. But I was not that woman, and trying to be her proved fruitless. Every one of my behaviors held potential implications for Veda. Was it okay to use a certain skin cream? Had I accidentally eaten unpasteurized cheese at a holiday party? Would sleeping on my back deprive her of oxygen? When Veda was born, I knew these kinds of questions would only multiply.

Fourteen minutes after Veda's arrival in the world, a postpartum nurse appeared at my bedside. It was time for my daughter to eat, she said, giving me a warm smile. The nurse gently scooted Veda up on my chest, then guided her nose and mouth toward the source of milk. My eyes focused on Veda, and I held my breath in anticipation.

By the time Veda was born, in 2019, I had already spent five years as a sociology graduate student researching the trials and tribulations of feeding children. That work, combined with countless conversations among friends and family about the challenges of breastfeeding, meant that I was braced for this moment. I expected nothing to be easy about feeding my daughter, now or in the future. Today I'd struggle with nursing a baby. In a year, I'd navigate a toddler's pickiness. In a decade, I'd face a teenager's love of fast food. When it came to food, the road ahead, as far as I could see, was anything but smooth.

Her skin glued to mine, Veda could barely open her eyes. I tracked her closely as she sniffed around. Then the nurse craned Veda's head back, and my daughter's tiny pink mouth opened. I watched her head fling forward as she clamped down on my breast and began to drink.

Thank God. I exhaled, feeling more relief than happiness. That nursing was physically painful was completely irrelevant.

My daughter was eating. And if she was eating, that meant she was fine. Great, even. For a moment, I felt satisfied. I was ensuring Veda's well-being. I was a good mom.

This was the first of many moments over the coming days, weeks, months, and years during which I would hold my breath. My husband, Ansu, also felt ownership for Veda's well-being, but biology significantly raised the stakes for me. As the parent using my own body to literally grow our daughter every single moment of every single day, I often felt like I had no respite from my responsibility for her.

Society has only reinforced my maternal sense of accountability for Veda. One particularly fraught setting for me — where I often feel reminded most viscerally of this accountability — has been our pediatrician's office. During those office visits, my daughter's height, weight, and body mass index (BMI) is fastidiously monitored to track her nutrition and development. On Veda's third day of life, Ansu and I brought her in for a routine checkup. In the exam room, we undressed her, fumbling like the new parents we were as we pulled her green-and-white-striped onesie up over her head and removed her diaper. Gingerly, Ansu placed her on the scale to be weighed.

"Let's see how good of a job Mom is doing," the nurse said cheerily, turning the scale on.

In that moment, my heart sank.

I knew the medical questions that lay behind the nurse's casual comment, and I assumed her intentions were good. I felt confident that she wasn't trying to single me out or place an added weight on my shoulders. She wanted to know how much Veda had been eating. She wanted to see whether my daughter had gained any ounces since being discharged from the hospital. These were reasonable questions about a newborn's development. But these were not the questions the nurse had asked. Instead, she had conveyed a very different message to me — one that made clear that I was only as good a mother as the number on that scale revealed. My daughter's body, I now understood, was feedback about my parenting.

Food is foundational. We eat multiple times a day from the day we are born to the day we die. To eat is to live. By extension, to feed others is to provide the means for them to survive and thrive. When parents feed their children, they act on an almost primal instinct to nourish their kids physically and emotionally. As a parent, to feed your children well is to succeed; to feed them poorly or to struggle to feed at all is to fail.

This book is about feeding families and the weight that bears on parents from all walks of life. Feeding, like any act of love, is both challenging and fulfilling. There are moments of frustration, triumph, and comic relief. But in this time and place—America in the twenty-first century—feeding has become both an extremely difficult task and a high-stakes parenting endeavor. Parents today feed their children against a national backdrop of mounting inequalities in wealth and health; a food environment increasingly saturated with sugar, salt, and fat; rising rates of childhood and adult obesity; and an insidious national discourse that emphasizes personal over social responsibility. This broader context shapes the obstacles parents today must overcome to fill kids' stomachs. It also showcases parents' creativity and devotion.

What parents feed their kids—and what gets eaten within families—also has profound implications for society at large. All of us were once kids ourselves. Most of us grew up within a family. That family may have taken different shapes—with one or two parents, with few or multiple generations, with or without siblings—but whatever the particulars, the food practices of our childhoods have had ripple effects extending into our adulthoods. As kids, we learned—either through explicit conversation or by observation—what and how to eat. We learned what constitutes a meal, what's "healthy" and "unhealthy," what foods are meant for daily consumption and what foods are reserved for special occasions. Our childhood diets cultivated our taste buds, familiarizing us with certain flavors and cultural traditions. Whether we identify today with what we ate as kids—whether we eat the same things our parents ate or whether we've paved new dietary paths for ourselves—what we saw, touched, smelled, and tasted as kids affects what we consume now. What we learned about nourishing ourselves then affects how we nourish ourselves today. And all of these lessons influence how we then nourish the next generation. While this is a book about how parents feed their kids, its stories, lessons, and relevance extend to every single one of us.

This book is a work of nonfiction. It is the product of years of ethnographic research on families' diets, most of which I conducted as a doctoral student in sociology at Stanford University. The people, places, and events I describe are real.

I carried out this research with the approval of Stanford University's institutional review board, an organizational body that oversees and protects the rights and welfare of people who participate in research studies. Everyone I spoke with consented to be part of a scientific study and all were made fully aware that their perspectives would be anonymously reported in journal articles and, potentially, a book. To safeguard the privacy and ensure the anonymity of my research participants, I replaced their real names with pseudonyms and altered any details that could help identify them, like the particular suburbs they lived in or the companies they worked for. I promised participants anonymity first and foremost for their own protection. But this promise also granted them the freedom to speak candidly without fear of one day having their identities disclosed.

To represent my research participants and to reconstruct events and conversations as accurately as possible, I used thousands of pages of field notes, interview transcripts, e-mails, and text records. From this extensive documentation I have edited quotations for length and, when absolutely necessary, clarity. I kept these edits as minimal as possible to allow the richness and diversity of individuals' voices and personalities to shine through. The families that participated in my research brought incredible generosity, candor, and vulnerability to our interactions. My aim here is to bring their experiences, struggles, and triumphs to life as truthfully and empathetically as possible.

"What's your goal with all this?" Joaquin Vargas, a stay-at-home father of two, asked me one afternoon. Joaquin was one of the first parents I interviewed for my research. Two cups of tea between us, refilled after almost two hours spent discussing his family's diet, Joaquin was curious to know whether he'd ever hear of me and my research again. Other parents echoed Joaquin's question. What was the point of all this work?

It's a question I'd often asked myself as well. At first, my principal goal was to contribute to social science research, an objective typically achieved through publishing articles in academic journals. I enjoyed—in fact, I still enjoy—much of this process. The deep and dynamic analysis of thousands of pages of interview transcripts and field notes, the grappling with sociological theory, and the challenge of ushering in data to substantiate an argument— accomplishing these tasks transformed me from a student into a sociologist. But I also felt called to reach broader audiences with my work and to move beyond the peer-review process to participate in a more public conversation. I began writing op-eds and doing radio and TV interviews about my research for outlets like the *Los Angeles Times,* Univision, and the Canadian Broadcasting Corporation. These led to further media appearances around the country and e-mails from physicians, researchers, students, parents, and activists with whom my research resonated. It was gratifying to engage with others about my work. In using my research to bring new data and ideas to public discourse, influence readers' views, and instigate conversation on issues I cared about, I felt, for the first time, that my work might actually help people.

These experiences gave me the answer to Joaquin's question. I wanted to write a book—*this* book—and a particular one at that. Books about food and diet are numerous. And I've spent years poring through them, carefully underlining passages, highlighting arguments, and scribbling my own notes in the margins. Having immersed myself in these texts for over a decade, I've noticed a shared trait: Books about food are often filled with insights or advice that makes us feel bad about how we are eating. They tell us that we should follow a plant-based diet or that our TV dinners are irreparably harming the planet. Because these books, informative as they may be, tend to be highly prescriptive, they can inadvertently make us more judgmental. They can encourage us to be increasingly critical of ourselves and others. This is a different kind of book. I hope you will find it short on judgment and long on empathy and evidence about the feeding challenges that unite and divide families across American society.

My professional role as a sociologist—and my own personal identities—are also woven into the story that follows. For years, I have written scientific articles partially in the passive voice: interviews were conducted, observations were made, data were analyzed. Such scientific norms have never bothered me, but they underscore how we scholars tend to abstract ourselves out of our research. Whether to sound more sophisticated or feign a veil of objectivity, we can make it seem as though we, as researchers, are nothing more than tools through which scientific truth is uncovered and knowledge is produced.

Yet try as we might, we are always a part of the research. As scientists, we cannot help but bring ourselves—how we identify, our past experiences, the biases we hold, the assumptions we'd rather not admit to—into the work we do. The research featured in this book exists only because I conducted it. I was the one who approached families at food banks, department stores, pharmacies, and gas stations. I designed the interview questions that asked parents about their kids' favorite snacks or whether they had ever not had enough to eat. I stood on my tiptoes to grab moms cartons of cereal from top supermarket shelves, chopped cherry tomatoes for salads, pulled frozen pizzas out of ovens, and sat beside kids at kitchen counters. I wrote up the field notes from my observations, analyzed the data over cups of tea at my own kitchen counter, and put the words to the pages you're reading now. All of these things made me part of the research that features in this book.

What follows here is my earnest attempt to be transparent about what it was like to be there and how I have come to understand those experiences. For a scientist, there can be safety in hiding behind a third-person voice and vulnerability in exposing one's own subjectivity through a first-person narrative. At the risk of criticism, I have chosen the latter. Throughout this book, I share not only what I saw but also what I thought, felt, questioned, and contended with over the years. My hope is that exposing this hidden part of the research process will bring clarity and context to you as a reader and help you understand how I arrived at my central arguments.

I brought to this research my own history and my own relationship with food. These reflect the multiple identities I hold as a biracial, second-generation South Asian American, highly educated millennial woman. As with most people's, my story with food began before I was born. What I know starts with my father, who grew up in India, and my mother, who was raised in both France and the United States. My parents' paths crossed in 1976 in New York City. That their first date was at a steak house aptly foreshadows meat as a dietary staple in our household.[1]

As in most American families, my mother was in charge of food at home. Her own childhood experiences shaped how she approached that task.

"I have great memories of food, and I have terrible memories of food," she explained to me one afternoon. Her fond memories were formed on both sides of the ocean. Some took place in Normandy, France's northwesternmost region, in her maternal grandmother's home. Normandy is filled with sparsely populated farmland: gently rolling hills dotted with cows and sheep, scattered houses framed by stone walls, and the occasional roadside stand selling fresh apple cider. My mother loved the food of Normandy; she delighted in warm baguettes with thick slabs of bright yellow butter, fatty soft cheeses, rich mashed potatoes, slow-cooked pork chops, and any and all vegetables my grandmother grew in the backyard. My mother similarly reveled in many of the dishes she ate during the summers that she spent in New York City. Her father, who was of Russian Jewish descent, would take her to Jewish delis in Manhattan, where they would enjoy pastrami sandwiches and dill pickles. On Saturdays, they would hop on the ferry to Staten Island for ice cream. Sunday nights meant Chinese food.

My mother's terrible memories of food were equally as sharp, centered mainly on the dishes her mother prepared. My grandmother, a petite Frenchwoman with an eye for order, placed severe restrictions around food. My mother was forbidden to eat American junk food. Portion sizes and snacks were limited, and my mother recalls feeling hunger pangs in the hours leading up to late dinners. But what my mother remembers most is being forced to eat foods that she loathed. Just the thought of a particular sour cream and green pepper salad is enough to make her shudder even now, sixty years later.

"I didn't want to do that to you," my mom told me, smiling. "I wanted you to love food."

For my mother, loving food meant having some say in what one ate. As a result, I grew up with very few dietary restrictions. My mom said no to some things—Twinkies and Cocoa Puffs, for instance—but yes to almost everything else. At home, we ate a smorgasbord of American, French, and Indian cuisines. There was a steady flow of bread, butter, and cheese in our kitchen. My mom prepared the pork chops and mashed potatoes of her youth, and she learned to cook new dishes like sausages and cabbage and salami-and-Gouda-cheese melts. We also devoured North Indian food. My father had fond memories of his childhood diet, which was rich in chicken, lamb, chana, and chapatis. "Everything was fresh, local, and delicately prepared," he told me. When he moved to Chicago, at twenty-three, my father quickly became a fan of American food's convenience, tastiness, and affordability. But because he missed the spices and flavors of his New Delhi childhood, he learned a few simple dishes, which he later taught my mother. Those were the dishes I grew up with: a ground lamb dish called keema, aloo gobi, dal, and well-buttered basmati rice with peas.

Looking back, what I remember most about my diet growing up is the freedom. I basically ate whatever I wanted. Many of those foods were nutritious. I adored peas and corn, bananas, roasted chicken, eggs, broccoli, and milk. But like many children's, my palate was primed for sugar and salt. There was nothing I wouldn't do for ice cream, cookies, and, most notably, hot dogs.

"For a year," my mother said, laughing, "you ate a hot dog for breakfast every morning." Hot dogs were delicious, but I also loved them because I was the one who chose and prepared them. They made me feel independent and capable. At six years old, I would carefully remove one link from the refrigerator, poke four holes in it with a fork, wrap it in a wet paper towel, and heat it for exactly one minute in the microwave. Then I'd set it inside a white, fluffy bun and scarf it down. While my breakfast habits became a running joke in the family—the particular irony being that I later became a vegetarian—I don't recall being chided or scolded for my food choices as a child.

My parents also treated us to inexpensive takeout on occasion, letting us choose Mexican, Chinese, or Italian food. Every time my dad picked me up from high-school volleyball practice,

I'd ask for a dollar milkshake, and he'd oblige. I drank soda and ate fast food.

"I didn't want to deliberately feed you junk," my mother told me when I asked her about it while writing this book. "But junk was always a part of what we ate."

"We're not saints!" my father added.

Age later brought changes to my own diet. At twenty, I began to eat more plants and fewer animals. Since then, I've had my fair share of dietary phases, pescatarianism and veganism among them. But for the most part, vegetarianism has been my home base for over a decade.

How I eat is a work in progress. I go through periods where my diet feels rich in whole foods; other times, I find myself leaning more on processed and prepared products. I genuinely love most vegetables and some fruits, but I will readily forgo them for a greasy slice of pizza or a generously iced wedge of carrot cake. I snack constantly, stockpile pastries, and notoriously oversalt my dinner. Cooking has long been a hobby of mine, but I don't know how to bake bread and I don't enjoy spending hours over a hot stove. Like most women in America, I've spent time worrying about my weight; I've gone through stretches where eating has been far less about enjoyment or health and far more about striving to meet societal standards of beauty. I consider myself extremely fortunate that I have always had enough money to buy not only the food I need but also the food I want.

Having now interviewed hundreds of people about how they eat, I feel like my relationship with food makes me part of the human race. It's a complicated, ever-changing bond. I control my portions one moment and eat my feelings the next. I've had phases of overeating and phases of undereating. I've dug my heels in on some food habits and worked patiently to change others. I use food for all kinds of purposes. Survival and satiation are part of it, but so are comfort, nostalgia, boredom, vanity, and celebration. I devour foods from my childhood because they remind me of happy moments, particular people, or special places. I eat foods to signal my membership in different communities or my various identities. And other foods end up in my stomach simply because I'm tired and impatient.

Balancing such priorities has shaped how I feed my daughter. As an infant, Veda drank breast milk and formula. She ate store-bought baby food. When she became a toddler, I fed her peas and oranges as well as Cheerios, pasta, and uthappam. Ansu and I care about how our daughter eats, but this concern is not the sole determinant of her diet. How we feed her on any given day depends in part on how tired we are and how much patience the three of us can muster during a meal. Sometimes Ansu and I have the bandwidth to negotiate with a stubborn toddler to get her to eat more of what we want her to; other times, Veda emerges from the meal victorious, the crumbs of her less preferred foods scattered across the dining-room floor. For me, as her mother, feeding Veda remains a source of both joy and conflict. Nourishing her feels at once natural and burdensome, as each spoonful I provide reminds me that I am on the hook for her. It reminds me that, try as I might, I cannot shake the responsibility that the nurse in my pediatrician's office assigned me years ago.

Let's see how good of a job Mom is doing.

To this day, this comment continues to ring in my ears. It reminds me of just how readily—casually, even—parents are put on trial for what and how much goes into their children's bodies.

The evidence summoned for these trials is often buttressed by metrics, like height, weight, and BMI, that assess whether children are being fed well, too much, or not enough. In the broadest sense, I support these measures as public health tools; limited as they may be, they also allow us to easily evaluate and compare kids' health across a population and identify precursors and symptoms of disease. In fact, the nutritional and health inequities revealed by such metrics provided one motivation for my research and this book. But these metrics have their limits and downsides. BMI, for instance, is a blunt diagnostic tool and an imprecise measure of health; calculated merely as a ratio of a person's weight to height, it does not take into account age, sex, or an individual's body composition, including how much of the weight comes from fat and how much from muscle. What's more, metrics like BMI can promote tunnel vision, focusing societal attention on kids' nutritional outcomes and leading us to over-look why there may be gaps between those outcomes and par-ents' efforts.[2]

Most parents I met as part of my research wanted to do what was best for their kids nutritionally and shared overlapping ideas of what "best" was. But they were dealt dramatically differ-ent hands to do so. Some parents had ample resources—enough time, a living wage, job security, stable housing, quality health care, social support, safe neighborhoods, and intergenerational wealth. Other parents lacked some or all of those resources. I saw how parents with fewer means struggled not only to get food on the table but also to maintain their dignity while being indicted for their kids' dietary outcomes. With inches and pounds as largely agreed-upon measures of kids' well-being, parents found—like I did—an upsetting truth: that their chil-dren's bodies served as an external signal of their worthiness as caregivers.

But scholarship and motherhood have opened my eyes to a different truth: While parenting is measured in outcomes, it's largely about effort. Much of this effort is hidden, performed daily by parents in a million unseen moments. A drawing by the artist Paula Kuka captures this reality nicely. On the left-hand side, under the words *What I Did,* she has drawn images of a mother changing one child's diaper, cooking for her children, consoling them, playing with them, nursing them, reading to them, dancing with them, and teaching them how to ride a bike.

On the right-hand side, under the words *What You Saw,* we see a mom pushing a stroller.

As a society, we see numbers and outcomes. And it's tempting to believe that there exists some linear relationship between parents' efforts and children's outcomes. Especially in America, a country largely rooted in the idea that people get what they strive for and deserve, it can be difficult to accept that the parents of kids with "poor" outcomes work just as hard as the parents of kids with "good" outcomes. It doesn't seem fair.

But just because something isn't fair doesn't make it any less true.

This book is an earnest attempt to expose and explore a largely hidden truth: that parents across society undertake sacrificial, complicated, and frustrating work to feed kids. Because the shape this work takes is context-dependent, it continually risks being overlooked, misunderstood, or, worst of all, condemned.

My hope is that by the time you reach this book's final pages, you'll have gleaned a deeper and more nuanced understanding of parents' nutritional efforts and obstacles. I also hope that you'll join me in asking how we as a society can move away from judging and critiquing parents to empathetically tackling their struggles. Rather than relentlessly heaping more responsibility and judgment onto parents' plates for what goes in kids' bodies, we can begin to regard kids' diets as a communal endeavor, one in which we all have a role to play. If we can accept this as our social and societal responsibility, then the question will no longer be: How should parents feed their kids? Rather, the question will become: How can we, as a society, ensure that parents—*all* parents—have the means necessary to nourish their children?

PART I

Divides

I often wondered: is it some kind of a trade-off? Do others have to lose so we can win?

— ZADIE SMITH, *SWING TIME*

CHAPTER 1

Diverging Destinies

On a sweltering summer afternoon, I sat in the back seat of a '91 Lexus sedan with the windows rolled down. It was July, and Silicon Valley was baking under a blazing sun and a cloudless sky. For the past two hours, I'd joined Nyah Baker and her fourteen-year-old daughter, Natasha, as they ran errands around town. My shoulder blades stuck to the car's black leather seats, and I looked forward to the brief moments of respite that came when we picked up speed and a breeze poured through the open windows. Behind the wheel, Nyah fiddled with the radio and settled on an R and B station; she turned up the volume and began to sing along. To her right, Natasha sank deep into the passenger seat, tapping away on her phone.

It had been just over a month since I'd started spending time with Nyah and her family. Driving with Nyah meant being constantly reminded that money was scarce. As we neared each intersection, she shifted the car into neutral, coasting the final feet to keep the gas light from coming on for just a little longer. All of July, Nyah had complained about the car's broken air-conditioning. Leather seats and hundred-degree weather didn't mix. But I knew it would be at least another month before Nyah had enough cash in hand to fix it.

Yet amid these recurring reminders that money was tight, there were rare moments when Nyah's worries temporarily subsided. In these moments, she almost seemed to forget that there was barely enough money for rent and utilities. One such moment came three hours into our outing, when Nyah and Natasha spotted the unmistakable green-and-white logo of a Starbucks café. A few minutes later, after a quick exchange of knowing glances, we were inside ordering at the counter. Nyah bought herself and Natasha two large Frappuccinos and offered to buy me one as well. "You can treat me next time," I assured her with a smile.

When the barista rang Nyah up, the number that flashed across the register caught me off guard. The drinks cost $10.80. An hour ago, I'd seen Nyah haggle with a cell phone agent to subtract one dollar off her monthly statement. Now she was spending double digits on two coffee-caramel milkshakes topped with whipped cream.

As we waited for the drinks at the counter, I found myself wondering why Nyah was putting her last few dollars for the month toward a pair of Frappuccinos rather than saving to repair the car's air-conditioning. This question begged a broader one, one that I'd found myself asking time and time again over the years I'd spent researching families' diets. What did these kinds of food purchases mean to moms like Nyah who were raising their kids in poverty? What would've been different about this exchange to moms with significantly more money in the bank?

That summer day, food's meaning to Nyah started to reveal itself to me. When the drinks popped up on the counter, I saw Nyah's face soften from worry to satisfaction. She handed Natasha a green straw and watched her daughter happily sipping her milkshake, taking extra care not to neglect the generous fluffy layer of whipped cream at the top. Sure, Nyah had put her last change toward the drinks. And sure, that money could have gone toward fixing the car or covering the overdue electricity bill. There wouldn't be money to fill the gas tank today, tomorrow, or the next day.

But for Nyah, the money had been well spent regardless. It

had gone to something much bigger: her daughter's momentary happiness. On the drive home from Starbucks, Nyah and Natasha savored their drinks. And, for the first time that day, no one seemed bothered by the lack of AC.

In 2014, I set out to research how American families eat. Between 2014 and 2016, I interviewed parents and children from seventy-five families and observed four families—including Nyah's—at length as they went about their daily lives eating and feeding. I also met with food-service workers, school administrators, and teachers, all of whom play a role in how families eat. My research introduced me to people from all walks of life. I met families living in gated communities, townhomes, trailer parks, and their cars. I spoke with dentists, cashiers, lawyers, janitors, software engineers, nurses, and sanitation workers. I came to know Black, Latinx, Asian, white, and multiracial families, single parents and married couples, fourth-generation American citizens and undocumented immigrants, stay-at-home caregivers and full-time workers. While I spent, on average, three to six hours with most of the families I interviewed, I spent months with the four that I followed in depth. Inside these families' homes, I poured bowls of cereal, reheated leftovers, sliced fruit on kitchen counters, and twirled spaghetti at dining-room tables. Outside their homes, I joined families as they navigated crowded supermarket aisles. I stood beside them in winding food-bank lines. I came to know the daily dietary rituals of the moms, dads, and kids, plus a few extended-family members and friends. I knew who took sugar and cream with their coffee and whether they dipped their fries in ketchup or ranch. Through it all, I learned how profoundly, at times paradoxically, families' circumstances shaped the way they ate.

In the "About This Project" section in the back of this book, I share the details of how this research came to be, including how I developed relationships with families, how I conceptualized my role as a researcher and confidante, how I wrestled with the ethical and practical issues that arose during my time embedded within families, and how everything I learned along the way changed me as a scholar and a human being. But it's worth touching on a few of these issues here.

Why did families let you spend so much time with them? Over the years, I've been asked this question in one form or another more times than I can count. There is no one-size-fits-all answer to it. Families' motivations for speaking to me—and, in some cases, spending months of their lives with me—varied. Certainly, some parents signed their families up for the money; sixty dollars in compensation for an interview was a decent deal. And I provided the families I observed at length three hundred dollars for their time, which was not an insignificant sum. But money wasn't the sole driver behind families' decisions to participate in my research. Parents who didn't need the money agreed simply because they were curious about the research. Others did it because a friend referred them. Still others took pity on a graduate student in need of data for her dissertation.

Whatever the families' motivations for signing up, who I was and how I presented myself likely helped facilitate their participation. It helped that I was a woman in my twenties, since conducting interviews and observations involved my spending many hours alone with mothers and children. I found that moms were comfortable with letting me inside and allowing me to speak with their kids in private; they were even eager to know if I had kids myself. When they discovered the answer was no, some told me to reach out again when I became a mother—they'd be happy to share their wisdom with me then too. While I never reached out later for that particular purpose, I was struck by the sincerity and warmth most moms showed in opening their doors and their lives to me.

I enjoyed spending time with families. Most made me feel like I belonged, treating me like an insider rather than an intruder. They invited me to birthday parties and communions, introduced me to extended family and friends, and never let me pay for gas (no matter how many times I offered). But I was vigilant about not letting families' generosity confuse me. No matter how well I came to know a family, no matter how much they shared or how kindly they included me, I always remembered the truth—that I was no insider. Their lives were not mine, and I would always be a researcher documenting their stories. My role as a researcher also implied an ethical responsibility to do no harm; mistakenly believing that I could ever truly walk a mile in families' shoes had the potential to do real damage. Such a misguided notion could convince me that I understood their struggles personally, that just because I'd watched them experience those hardships, I knew those hardships too.

I did not. I do not. And instead of trying to, I strove to employ in my research approach what the Pulitzer Prize–winning author Isabel Wilkerson calls radical empathy. Radical empathy involves putting in the work "to educate oneself and to listen with a humble heart to understand another's experience from *their* perspective, *not* as we imagine *we* would feel."[1] Radical empathy demands that you accept the limits of your understanding, given who you are and the hand you've been dealt in life. Rather than trying to make sense of other people from your own perspective and lived experience, you must work to understand their experiences deeply, from their perspectives and lived experiences.

Radical empathy is a tall order, and I would never claim to have wholly succeeded at it. Like all human beings, I am prone to biases born of my own experiences that color how I make sense of everything I observe. But an awareness of these biases— and a continual commitment to questioning them—also positioned me to see what others might have missed when it came to families' diets. As families granted me the rare opportunity to walk beside them, I worked to grasp their worlds the way *they* saw and experienced them. In doing so, I gained a deeper, richer appreciation of the fuller contexts encompassing their lives. When it came to how families ate, choices that likely seemed strange from the outside appeared perfectly understandable. What society, the media, and scholars deemed irrational, irresponsible, or misguided began to make perfect sense to me. And I learned that nothing short of radical empathy is what I needed—what all of us need—to understand families' diets today, as well as the deeply entrenched inequalities that drive those diets apart.

Before embarking on this research, I knew a few important facts about the standard American diet, or SAD, as it's cheekily known. The American diet is "sad" because it's generally unhealthy. Despite how contentious discussions about what's healthy and unhealthy can feel, the nutrition community actually largely agrees about what constitutes a nutritious diet—and most Americans aren't eating it. Nutritious diets consist primarily of plant-based whole foods and are rich in fruits and vegetables, whole grains, low- or fat-free dairy, legumes, nuts, and seafood. They are low in red and processed meats, refined grains, and added sugar.[2]

Even the federal government agrees. Every five years, beginning in 1990, the U.S. Department of Agriculture has published the *Dietary Guidelines for Americans* (*DGA*). The *DGA* provides the public with food-based recommendations to meet their nutrient needs and help prevent diet-related chronic diseases.[3] To be fair, the *DGA* doesn't always promote optimal nutrition science, as food-and-beverage-industry lobbyists work their own interests into federal nutritional advice. But even with industry influence, the *DGA*'s recommendations broadly align with those of nutrition scientists. The *DGA* currently recommends that half one's plate should be fruits and vegetables, a quarter should be grains or starches, and a quarter should be protein; a meal should also include some low-fat dairy. These general dietary prescriptions allow ample room for personal choice, leaving it up to individuals to customize their diets with any combination of these foods.

But the majority of Americans don't follow these guidelines. Most fall short of meeting the *DGA*, and Americans consistently score poorly on measures assessing dietary health.[4] One commonly used diet-quality scale, the Healthy Eating Index, scores a person's diet quality from 0 (lowest quality) to 100 (highest quality). The average American diet earns a failing score of 59.[5] Three-quarters of Americans eat a diet low in vegetables, fruits, dairy, and oils and high in added sugars, saturated fats, and sodium. Fewer than one in ten Americans eat enough vegetables and fruits, and most consume too many calories each day.[6]

Like American adults, American kids aren't getting the nutrients they need. Slightly over half of children and two-thirds of adolescents eat a low-quality diet with too much sodium, too many processed foods, and too few vegetables.[7] On average, kids consume eighteen teaspoons — or just over seventy-one grams — of added sugar every day, making sugar one out of every seven calories they eat.

Sad as the American diet may be, it's actually improved modestly since the turn of the twentieth century, largely due to widespread nutrition-education efforts and food-safety advances. Between 2002 and 2012, the share of people in the United States eating an unhealthy diet fell from around 56 percent to under 46 percent. Americans have slowly started eating more whole grains, nuts, and seeds and consuming less meat (specifically beef and pork). They've also begun drinking fewer sugar-sweetened beverages. The statistics on children are similarly encouraging: in 1999, three-fourths of kids ate what is termed a low-quality diet; in 2016, just around half did so. Kids are also eating more whole grains, yogurt, and fruits and vegetables and drinking fewer sugar-sweetened beverages.

And yet these national dietary gains have not been shared equally across American society. Study after study has revealed nutritional inequalities across socioeconomic status and race and ethnicity in America.[8] Improvements in diet over the past decades have largely been concentrated among middle- and higher-income Americans. In particular, high-income Americans are now eating better than ever—more often swapping fruit juice for whole fruits, replacing refined grains with whole grains, and eating tons of nuts—while improvements among lower-income Americans have been much more modest. Such dietary strides have also been racially patterned; white people's diets have been steadily improving over time, while Black and Mexican-American individuals haven't experienced the same upward trends. Such inequities exist for both adults and children.[9]

These nutritional disparities are alarming because of just how much diets matter for our overall health and well-being. Unhealthy eating causes more than half a million deaths per year and is linked to multiple chronic diseases, including cardiovascular disease, high blood pressure, several types of cancer, and type 2 diabetes.[10] Today, an unhealthy diet is the leading contributor to mortality in the United States. What we eat has become, quite literally, a matter of life and death.

Because our diets have such profound implications, nutritional disparities help drive broader health disparities that disproportionately harm individuals already marginalized in American society—low-income communities and racial and ethnic minorities. Compared to high-income Americans, low-income Americans have greater rates of diet-related disease and shorter life spans. They are also five times more likely to report being in poor or fair health. People of color similarly bear the disproportionate burden of diet-related illness. Compared to white people, Black, Latinx, and American Indian individuals have higher rates of chronic disease and fewer years of life.[11] While the factors underlying socioeconomic and racial health disparities are multifaceted and complex, nutritional inequalities help perpetuate them over time and across generations.

Nutritional and health inequalities also tie into a much broader story of American inequality. Economically, inequality has long been on the rise, with the gap between the haves and have-nots becoming perhaps the most defining and consequential feature of contemporary life in the United States. While the rich have gotten much richer since the 1970s, nearly everyone else has seen their incomes stagnate or decline. The top 1 percent of earners' annual wages have grown by 135 percent over the past thirty years, but middle- and working-class wages have stagnated and declined, respectively. In 2015, the top 1 percent of families nationally made over twenty-six times as much as the bottom 99 percent.[12]

Inequality today is not only growing within generations; it also remains shockingly durable across them. This fact stands in stark contrast to the American Dream, which promises that hard work and opportunity will lead to a more prosperous life, if not for oneself, then at least for one's children. The American Dream delivered for many kids born in the middle of the twentieth century—more than 90 percent of Americans born in 1940 were earning more at the age of thirty than their parents had earned at the same age. But today, that American Dream has become a mirage. Only half of kids born in 1980 earned more at the age of thirty than their parents had earned at that age. Kids born to affluent parents since the 1980s are most likely to grow up to be affluent, while the children of the poor are more likely to remain poor their entire lives.[13] These economic inequalities are neither natural nor inevitable but the direct consequence of American social policy that has eroded the social safety net over time, depressed real wages, and largely avoided instituting strong family policies that support child-rearing and caretaking.[14]

Economic inequalities are intimately intertwined with racial and ethnic inequalities, leading people of color to be disproportionately represented among those with lower incomes and less education. Stark and persistent racial disparities in Americans' economic well-being reflect a legacy of systemic, structural racism throughout American history. In particular, enduring, deeply rooted racial discrimination in many forms—including in education, housing, hiring, and pay practices—has generated persistent earnings gaps between white individuals and those of color. Over the past fifty years, the racial income gap has not budged. In 1968, shortly after the passage of the Civil Rights Act, the median Black family income was 57 percent that of whites. In 2016, it was 56 percent. But the starkest racial divides are in household wealth, reflecting centuries of white privilege that have made it particularly difficult for people of color to achieve economic security. Today, the average Black family with children holds just one cent of wealth for every dollar that the average white family with children holds.[15]

These intersecting economic and racial inequities mirror America's nutritional divides; as the country's most socioeconomically and racially privileged draw farther and farther ahead, the rest are left farther and farther behind. Nowhere was this more apparent than during the COVID-19 pandemic. In my final days of writing this book, SARS-CoV-2, the novel coronavirus, spread across the globe. As it did, domestic rates of unemployment, poverty, food insecurity, and hunger soared in the United States, with Black, Latinx, American Indian, and low-income communities hit the hardest. These same communities also experienced disproportionate rates of COVID-19 infections, hospitalizations, and deaths.

Researchers attributed these severe disease outcomes and disparities to multiple causes. For one, more low-income people and people of color had jobs that qualified them as essential workers; they had less ability to social distance or work from home, and this increased their risk of viral exposure. Furthermore, these groups faced longstanding barriers to health insurance, health-care facilities, and equitable treatment by health-care providers, which increased the virus's harmful, often lethal, impact. But worse viral outcomes were also associated with the kinds of diet-related chronic diseases—such as heart disease and type 2 diabetes—disproportionately affecting low-income communities and communities of color. In this way, the inequalities largely responsible for driving nutritional disparities across race and class also helped fuel the virus's disproportionate impact on America's most vulnerable groups. As these communities fared astonishingly worse overall than their wealthier, whiter counterparts, the inequalities that have long permeated American society grew more visible than ever before in modern history.[16]

I was first exposed to these inequalities at nine years old. It was 1995, and my family had just begun fostering children. Over the next five years, four foster children—two special-needs, medically fragile babies and two elementary-school siblings—came to live with us through the State of Arizona's foster-care system.

I observed and interacted with this foster-care system largely within the four walls of my family's home in Tucson. I knew from an early age that this system was infinitely bigger than anything my eyes could show me. I could see my foster siblings' clothes, watch their facial expressions, hear their intonations, share their favorite foods, and listen to their native tongues. I could count endless appointments, court hearings, and meetings with medical specialists, school counselors, social workers, and extended family. I could observe my parents—who were willingly fostering children, who had *chosen* to be a part of the system—constantly struggling to work within and push back against it.

This experience left me feeling deeply conflicted about foster care and the American safety net. The foster-care system was brimming with ambiguities and contradictions. At times, its institutions appeared to work in kids' interests, temporarily removing them from abusive or unsafe environments. It offered food, shelter, and care when children needed them most. In some cases, I felt that the system had done right by kids in placing them under our roof. And every so often, happy endings unfolded, like my foster brother's reunion with his biological mother following her completion of a rehabilitation program.

But other times, the outcomes weren't so clearly positive. Some of the kids who ended up in foster care, I suspected, might well have been better off staying out of it. When the system tore kids away from their parents, separated them from siblings, and shuffled them from home to home with no end in sight, it wasn't clear that kids' well-being was the administration's highest priority. From where I was sitting, the harms to a kid in the system could potentially outweigh the benefits.[17]

As I grew up, observing the system's gaps and shortcomings fueled my desire to know more. I wanted to understand what had happened to my foster siblings *before* they showed up at our front door. I was aware that my siblings' stories often involved experiences of deep poverty, unemployment, parental incarceration, substance use, and sexual, physical, or emotional abuse. But what had caused my siblings to encounter those circumstances? What forces were shaping my siblings' lives, and how did those forces relate to the ones shaping mine?

My foster (and, eventually, adopted) brother Josh helped me explore these questions. I first met Josh on a February afternoon in a hospital neonatal intensive care unit. Josh was born three months premature, weighing in at just under two pounds, and the first minute of his life forever changed the rest of it: sixty oxygen-deprived seconds created the physical and cognitive disabilities he'd bear forever, including cerebral palsy, microcephaly, and a host of developmental delays.

Quickly following Josh's birth, the State of Arizona severed the legal rights of his biological mother, Tracy. At the time, Tracy was herself a child at seventeen years old. While the state may have deemed her a perpetrator, she had also been a victim, bearing scars of persistent childhood neglect, domestic abuse, and her own harrowing experiences in the foster-care system.

Even though Tracy was without legal parental rights, my

parents were resolute about offering her the chance to be a part of Josh's life. She would always be his mother, even if the circumstances prevented her from assuming the caregiving role that status usually entailed. Until she passed away, at the age of thirty-two, Tracy was an important part of Josh's life and of our lives too. We saw her consistently for decades. She sat at our dinner table. She attended Josh's school graduations and birthday parties. During his multiple hospital stays, Tracy visited him. When Tracy gave birth years later to a second son, Jeremy, we all met Josh's younger half brother.

Tracy's life imprinted on mine. She and I were eight years apart. In another world, she could have been my big sister, my babysitter, or my cool older neighbor. She might have swung by my neighborhood lemonade stand or told me all about what to expect in high school.

But in this world, she was none of those things. Tracy and I had been born into dramatically different circumstances: Tracy into poverty, me into the middle class. I lived in a physically and psychologically safe home and neighborhood. Her childhood home had been anything but. The gulf between our experiences felt greater than our difference in age.

Without Josh, my path would almost certainly not have crossed with Tracy's. But with Josh, our lives were intimately intertwined. As the mother of my brother, she was, in some ways, my family. And observing Tracy—her diffident smile, her kind eyes, her high-waisted jeans—I found myself often considering the fact that her life could have been mine. Why hadn't I been born Tracy, and Tracy born me?

Through my foster siblings, I observed firsthand other lives I could have led, other circumstances in which I could have been raised. How had I ended up here and they ended up there? The facts were these: For a moment, we all existed in the same world. We lived under the same roof, slept in the same rooms, shared the same clothes. We sat around the same dinner table, attended the same schools, watched the same TV shows. But the similarities that bound us in those moments were, well, momentary. They were completely contingent on a system that temporarily tethered us together. I knew that because of the different worlds from which we had come and to which we would ultimately return, our destinies would eventually diverge. I came to understand, as deeply as a child can, that my life and my future were largely sculpted by one lucky, arbitrary chance—to whom and where I'd been born.

Years later, as a doctoral student researching social inequality, I often thought back to these early interactions with the foster-care system. I'd reflect on the inequities I'd seen shape my life and those of my foster siblings, and I'd connect what I was learning in lectures and articles to what I'd beheld with my own eyes. During this period, I found myself grappling with one particular aspect of inequality that I'd observed as a child but that didn't seem to feature prominently in sociological research.

That aspect was food.

For years, I witnessed the interplay between food and inequality in the foster-care system. I saw how deeply rooted inequalities affected my foster siblings' and my diets and how those diets had far-reaching consequences for our health and well-being. I'd fed some of my foster siblings through feeding tubes and watched while others hoarded cans of soup under their beds. I observed how my siblings wanted and begged for foods unfamiliar to me and how my own cravings could similarly perplex them. I witnessed how, when everything was constantly changing around these kids—people, houses, pets, furniture—food could become a rare source of stability and refuge.

I had seen how the human need to eat unites us, but the way that each of us meets that need pushes us farther apart. Now, what I wanted to uncover was *how*.

CHAPTER 2

Families in an Age of Inequality

One summer afternoon in 2014, in the cluttered, windowless office at Stanford University where I spent most of my days as a doctoral student, I sat at my desk reviewing the latest research on nutritional inequality in America. I was searching for information about its causes.

One epidemiological article reported that, from 2000 to 2010, diet disparities between rich and poor Americans had not only persisted but widened.[1] I scrolled through the article on my laptop, speed-reading until I reached the conclusion. Here was where I thought the authors might discuss what was causing these growing disparities.

The conclusion's first sentences were encouraging. "There are several potential explanations for the disparities across income levels," the authors began. My office chair creaked as I leaned forward, ready for answers to my questions. The authors proposed two.

The first was price. They explained that "price is a major determinant of food choice, and healthful foods generally cost more than unhealthful foods in the United States." The second was geographic access to healthy foods. "Access to healthful foods also contributes to income-related disparities," the authors wrote. "Low-income households are less likely to own a car and thus may have limited access to supermarkets that sell healthful foods."

From there, the authors seamlessly and speedily moved on to other topics, including their study's strengths and limitations and directions for future research. I closed the laptop and my eyes for a moment.

Is that really it? I wondered. My confusion was exceeded only by my skepticism. Was nutritional inequality completely explained by the fact that healthy food was more expensive and farther away from lower-income folks than wealthier ones? Were price and proximity *the* primary factors shaping how Americans ate?

Trying to set my skepticism aside momentarily, I decided to take a walk and clear my head. I stuffed my phone and keys into the back pocket of my jeans, shut my office door behind me, and descended a flight of stairs to the ground floor.

Outside, the air was still, and the sun filtered through palm trees onto the pavement. My mind wandered to a chilly autumn afternoon in Manhattan. The year was 1990. I was five years old. After my mom picked me up from kindergarten, we took the bus to my favorite place in the entire world: a bagel shop one block from our apartment. Inside, the air was warm and smelled of toasted bread, garlic, and onion. My mom ordered us two bagels—one plain bagel with cream cheese for me, one sesame bagel with butter for her. I hung my coat on a chair back as the plastic red baskets with our bagels popped up at the pickup counter. My mom grabbed them and set them down in front of us. The steam and scent rose toward my nose. I looked at my mom, admiring her easy smile and long, auburn hair tied loosely in a low ponytail. Nothing could beat my favorite food at my favorite place with my favorite person.

Now, as I weaved my way through campus, dodging students biking to and from class, a pang of nostalgia hit. I longed to be back in that moment—to stare across a wobbly wooden table at my mother as we bit into steaming bread and licked cream cheese or butter from our fingers. This was not the first time I'd felt this way. As a first-year college student, homesick and lonely, I had trudged in subzero Chicago temperatures to a sandwich shop to enjoy a toasted sesame bagel slathered in butter. While I was still a plane ride away, each bite made me feel just a tiny bit closer to my family.

The farther I walked, the deeper in thought I sank. I meditated on a simple truth that so many of my life's most salient memories were connected to food. From my childhood in Arizona, I could still hear the sizzle of eggs frying in a pan on Sunday mornings in my family's kitchen. I could smell the toasted cumin and coriander in steaming bowls of dal I devoured in my grandparents' New Delhi home. I could taste the chocolate chip cookies my older brother and I fought over in high school. In college, I reveled in the newfound freedom of all-you-can-eat dining-hall buffets. I packed dried cereal into paper cups and smuggled them back to my dorm room as snacks for late-night study sessions. When I moved into my first shared apartment, I baked frozen pizzas and roasted broccoli florets in the oven. I savored what felt like adulthood as I prepared breakfasts of Greek yogurt, granola, and sliced banana. After college, living in Germany, I enjoyed slowly perusing the aisles of unfamiliar supermarkets and sampling new foods. I felt a part of German culture as I ordered my Franzbrötchen, a north German cinnamon bun, from the local bakery. Later, when I settled in California as a graduate student, I loved cooking barefoot while listening to my music of choice in my tiny studio apartment. After dinner, I ate cookie dough ice cream with a long spoon out of the carton, the freezer door open.

So many foods embedded in so many of my memories. Some of these foods I no longer ate; others remained staples in my diet. What united them all, though, was that they felt like a part of me—etched into who I'd been and who I'd become. They all *meant* something to me. Fried eggs meant home, casseroles comfort and family, Franzbrötchen adventure, and frozen pizzas freedom. Some made me feel warmth, comfort, and joy; others transported me back to grief or loneliness.

I eventually found my way back to the office and plopped

myself down at my desk. I remained engrossed in thought about food's connections to certain places, people, and feelings in my life. How did those connections shape *my* food choices? As the article's authors had noted, what was both financially affordable and geographically available had in part influenced my dietary decisions. I didn't buy foods priced beyond my graduate-student budget, and I only had the time and energy to travel so far to eat (although I understood that being a full-time student without caregiving responsibilities granted me a unique amount of scheduling flexibility). But beyond price and proximity, my choices were shaped by what food meant to me and how it made me feel. I ate for pleasure and connection. I ate to satiate and to remember. I ate to show affection and to rejoice in celebration. I ate to signal who I was, where I came from, and what I believed in.

But was I alone in attaching such significance to food? I didn't think so.

This hunch catapulted me into years of research on families' diets. My goal was to understand how families ate and how their different circumstances shaped the food they put in their bodies. I wanted to know whether price and proximity were the only things that mattered and, if not, what else factored in. Through it all, I learned that the contexts within which families live shape their physical, logistical, financial, and psychological access to eating healthy food. But families' disparate contexts also fuel dietary inequalities by affecting something even more fundamental. They affect the very meaning of food itself. Food's different meanings to families across society, I came to see, are central to the story of nutritional inequality today. And I learned that only by understanding these meanings will we have a shot at reducing the inequities that drive our diets apart.

For my research I interviewed one hundred sixty parents and kids and observed four families in depth. Because adolescence is a particularly vulnerable nutritional period—kids' diet quality generally declines when they become teenagers—I focused on families with teenagers, although many also had younger children and a few had young adults who lived at home.

All of the families lived, as I did, in the San Francisco Bay Area, one of the most unequal places in the country. Over the past thirty years, incomes for Bay Area families in the top ninetieth percentile have grown by 60 percent while those for families in the bottom tenth percentile have edged up a mere 20 percent. Today, the ninetieth-percentile earners bring in around $400,000 a year, while the bottom tenth make just over $30,000.[2]

The Bay Area owes its skyrocketing inequality to the social and economic changes that accompanied the growth of new industries such as the tech sector. Bigger incomes at the top increased the cost of living for everyone, including low- and middle-income earners, whose wages largely stagnated. Sky-high rents and the vanishing possibility of home ownership have driven low-income families and communities of color from its inner to its outer reaches, or out of the region altogether.

Yet even within the wealthiest areas, concentrated affluence and poverty coexist. In every single Bay Area county, the number of families living in poverty has grown since the 1980s. In San Mateo County, where I rented an apartment my final year of graduate school, I saw extended families living in their RVs just a stone's throw away from exquisitely landscaped gated mansions. Tech moguls drove their Teslas down streets lined with public housing. Twenty-something data scientists making six figures ordered coffee from single mothers working two jobs to make ends meet.

While the Bay Area's juxtaposition of affluence and poverty feels extreme, it is also increasingly characteristic of American life. In an age of rising inequality, the region has been a trendsetter, not an outlier. Today, America is looking more and more like the Bay Area: increasing residential segregation, a hollowing of the middle class, and growing financial hardship among the poor. While the families I met all lived in the Bay Area, they tell a very all-American story. They also showcase the diversity of that story, hailing from different socioeconomic, racial, and cultural backgrounds.

In most families, I almost always spent time with the moms. Moms were the ones who generally responded to my calls, set up interviews, and hosted me when I came over. Dads were sometimes, but not always, present. There were exceptions to this general rule; I met a handful of families whose fathers, some of whom were stay-at-home parents, took the lead on food. But these cases were rare in my study, just as they are across the country. Despite societal gains in gender equality at home over the past century, American moms today remain families' primary caregivers. Moms still do more of the work of raising kids and managing homes, spending more time each day on their children and having less leisure time for themselves compared to dads. In 2016, mothers spent a weekly average of fourteen hours on childcare; dads spent eight hours. Moms devoted eighteen hours a week to housework; dads put in ten hours a week.

The statistics are even starker when it comes to who does the feeding. In four out of five families headed by married, heterosexual couples, mothers are the primary food providers. Even when both parents work outside the home, mothers continue to do most of the foodwork. They grocery shop, cook and clean up, and pack lunches and snacks. They also shoulder feeding's cognitive and emotional labor, including meal planning, worrying about what family members should be eating, and navigating and negotiating different food preferences and allergies. When it comes to cooking, moms spend three times as much time on meal preparation every day as dads, clocking sixty-eight minutes versus twenty-three minutes.[3] The families I met generally followed this very gendered pattern, with moms assuming the vast majority of responsibility for shopping, prepping, and cooking. Some of these moms enjoyed or took pride in this responsibility, while others loathed or resented it. Regardless, all of them did the work.

For this book, I debated how best to show how this food-related work played out across families. How could I both showcase the shared experiences binding moms while also revealing important differences between them? I landed, ultimately, on an imperfect solution. In the following pages, I delve most deeply into the lives of the four families I observed extensively while interweaving others' stories in. Doing so allows me to share details of families' experiences while also highlighting their heterogeneity.

The four families I spent the most time with came from varied educational, economic, and ethno-racial backgrounds. The Bakers were a Black family living below the federal poverty line; the Williamses were a working-class white family just above it; the Ortegas were a middle-class Latinx family; and the Cains were an affluent white family.[4] These families' stories do not represent all families that share their socioeconomic or racial/ethnic characteristics. The Ortegas don't exemplify every middle-class Latinx family, nor are the Cains a universal depiction of all affluent white families. Each family's diet was uniquely theirs. At the same time, their experiences highlight particular dietary challenges, feelings, and meanings shared by families with overlapping situations.

Below, I introduce the Bakers, Williamses, Ortegas, and Cains before delving into their diets. While raising their children under dramatically different circumstances, the moms in each family were united by their devotion to their kids and their desire to use food to do right by them.

The Bakers

I first met Nyah Baker at her home on a damp, overcast January afternoon. Two days prior, I'd interviewed her sister Dominique, who had pointed me in Nyah's direction for another interview.

"She needs that sixty bucks," Dominique said with a chuckle as she pulled out her phone to text her sister. Forty seconds later,

Dominique told me I could drive over to Nyah's for the interview. Given that it often took weeks or even months to schedule interviews, Nyah's availability caught me off guard. But I'd soon learn that what Nyah lacked in money she made up for in time.

A lecture on campus pulled me back to Stanford that afternoon, so Nyah and I scheduled our meeting for two days later. Nyah lived just ten minutes down the road from Dominique on a wide, peaceful residential street lined with Buicks and Fords and sparsely dotted with trees. Nyah was one of five million Americans living in Section 8 housing. The Section 8 Housing Choice Voucher Program is a form of government rent assistance through which private landlords can rent to qualified low-income families at a market rate; the federal vouchers cover some or all of the family's rent, while the family takes care of the rest. Many of Nyah's neighbors were also voucher recipients. When Nyah moved in eight years ago, she paid $87 a month in rent. Now, she was paying $603. But Nyah knew that she was lucky; most Americans don't live in public or voucher-subsidized housing, and three out of four who qualify for assistance don't actually receive any.[5]

Nyah loved her three-bedroom house with its spacious garage that she'd converted into a second living room. For the past eight years, it had been home to her and her two younger daughters: Mariah, now sixteen years old, and Natasha, now fourteen. Nyah's eldest, twenty-four-year-old Latoya, lived in Arizona with her husband and their son.

The afternoon I met Nyah, she opened the front door dressed in black sweatpants and a neon-green hoodie. Her long, black, braided hair was pulled into a tight bun atop her head, with a leopard-patterned headband to keep the flyaways at bay. Across one collarbone, the word *family* was tattooed in black cursive.

Nyah and I hit it off instantly. She had a straight-shooting candor and self-assuredness that made conversation easy. You could talk to Nyah for an hour and think it was twenty minutes. Part of what made the time fly was Nyah's disarming humor, an effortless blend of self-deprecation and lighthearted teasing. With food, as with other topics, Nyah was authentic and unabashed. "I've got nothing to hide," she told me the first day we met. She meant it.

Over time, I grew to be in awe of Nyah. Despite enduring countless traumas, she approached life and looked to the future with a seemingly bottomless well of hope, ingenuity, and guts.

Nyah was born in Georgia; when she was seven, her mom fled with her and her four siblings to escape a physically abusive domestic situation. They found refuge in Northern California, near Nyah's maternal grandmother. But soon after arriving on the West Coast, Nyah's mom got caught up in a bad crowd, spiraling into drug addiction and leaving Nyah and her siblings largely on their own. Nyah had to grow up fast. She took care of her two younger sisters, one of whom was Dominique, shielding them from their mother's addiction and sexually predatory male relatives and family friends.

"I had to play the role of a mom at a young age," Nyah recalled as we sat at her kitchen table. When Nyah turned fourteen, she became a mom herself. After years of repeated sexual assaults by her uncle, Nyah discovered she was pregnant. When Latoya was born, Nyah was forced to drop out of school to care for her daughter.

"The only way I knew how to survive and to feed my baby," Nyah said with a sigh, "was to go out and sell my body." Nyah's teenage years were dark, not only because of this but also because of her drug and alcohol addictions. But when Nyah turned twenty, two wonderful things happened. First, she got clean. Second, she met Darius, who would later give her Mariah and Natasha. Things were good for a while, even though money continued to be tight and the two had their issues. For the most part, Nyah was happy. But when Darius died of a stroke a decade later, Nyah was left alone with the two girls. Now, Nyah was raising them as a single mom. She was one of twenty-one single mothers I met during my research and one of over nine million single mothers in the United States.

I met both Mariah and Natasha that first afternoon too. Natasha, with thick black cornrows, a white gap-toothed smile, and a red T-shirt, waved hello from the couch, where she spent most of the afternoon tapping away on her phone. Mariah, in a black yoga tank top and leggings, her hair in a high bun with wandering strands down her cheeks, sauntered in and out of the house over the course of two hours. At one point, she carried a brown bag from McDonald's filled with two cheeseburgers and a sixteen-ounce soda for her sister.

Mariah and Natasha were sweet-tempered, soft-spoken girls. They were also best friends. Nyah saw herself in both of them. Mariah was an easy kid, Nyah told me, as Nyah herself had been. "She's not all wild and stuff." Nyah beamed. "She's not into the stuff that most kids her age are into." Natasha had Nyah's sense of humor. She was the comedian of the family, a tomboy with a bright smile. "I never had a boy, so she's like my son." Nyah laughed. "Crazy, sexy, and cute all in one."

The three got on well. The girls helped Nyah host neighborhood barbecues, where they would grill steaks and prepare bowls of potato salad. In the evenings, the three of them would immerse themselves in movie marathons, repeating their favorite romantic comedies from Nyah's extensive pirated-DVD collection. Nyah's pride in her girls was always on display. Mariah and Natasha were going to do better than she had. They were going to finish high school. Already, Nyah's eldest daughter, Latoya, had broken the cycle of becoming an early-teen mom. She'd waited until she was seventeen to get pregnant, Nyah explained.

I also came to know Nyah's boyfriend, Marcus, a lanky, gruff man in his forties who concealed his skin-and-bones physique under oversize T-shirts and baggy shorts. Marcus often hung around in front of the house. A neighborhood mechanic, he spent most afternoons working on his own car, a worn blue van permanently parked at the foot of Nyah's driveway. Nyah loved Marcus deeply, but his limited ability to contribute financially coupled with his heavy alcohol use left Nyah feeling profoundly alone. She couldn't depend on him or anyone else to help support her and her girls economically, emotionally, or psychologically. Nyah's experience reflected the economic reality in America for single moms, a third of whom are raising their children in poverty, nearly five times more than married-couple families.

"It's like I'm in this all by myself," Nyah told me one morning as Jerry Springer flashed across the garage TV screen. "I'm the one taking care of the bills and making sure we keep a roof over our heads, food in our mouths, clothes on our backs."

For years, Nyah had made good money as a cleaning lady. She worked long hours scrubbing toilets, mopping hardwood floors, and sanitizing sink basins. Thirteen dollars an hour wasn't much, but it added up over fifty or sixty hours each week. But the year I met Nyah, she was confronting a set of disabling health conditions that took her out of the workforce. At thirty-nine, Nyah felt that she was facing the challenges of someone double her age. She was a type 2 diabetic, had hypertension, and was awaiting a hysterectomy to address a painful, debilitating overgrowth of uterine fibroids. She had a slipped disk in her back and relentless, dull pain in her joints. Mentally, Nyah struggled with depression and anxiety.

Nyah's health conditions struck me, first and foremost, as the consequence of weathering. The weathering hypothesis, which was first proposed by the public health scholar Arline Geronimus in 1992, argues that the constant stress of racism—for Black women in particular—leads to premature biological aging and poor health outcomes. Geronimus proposed, and mounting research since has corroborated, that Black women's health deteriorates in early adulthood as a consequence of cumulative exposure to socioeconomic adversity, political marginalization, and the lived experience of ongoing racism and discrimination.[6]

Together, Nyah's health conditions made working impossible. Nyah had no choice but to rely on government support to make ends meet. She felt ashamed of that fact. It was not who she was. That shame was matched only by the financial stress she felt daily. Nyah had filed for disability benefits months ago, but she had yet to see any checks arrive in the mail.

In the meantime, Nyah made ends meet by constructing both a formal and an informal safety net for herself. Her income consisted mostly of monthly sixteen-hundred-dollar Supplemental Security Income (SSI) payments she received for her daughters' learning disabilities. That covered some of her expenses, including the highly subsidized rent of $603, utilities, cable, cell phones, and gas for her car. Nyah was also resourceful; she recycled beer cans, borrowed cash from her aunt, took out payday loans, and pawned her jewelry. When paying the bills demanded another hustle, Nyah took temporary employment as a sex worker. Nyah had no savings and thousands of dollars in credit card debt that she knew would never be paid off.

The Williamses

"It takes a village," Dana Williams told me as we sat at her kitchen table one swampy afternoon in early June. Like Nyah, Dana was a single mom raising two daughters: thirteen-year-old Madison and five-year-old Paige. The Williamses' eight-hundred-square-foot, two-bedroom apartment was a ten-minute walk from Dana's childhood home. Over the past few decades, the placid, residential area had changed significantly, transforming from a working-class white neighborhood of front yards displaying American flags to a community of primarily first- and second-generation Mexican-American families.

At four foot eleven with short, flat-ironed brown hair and a face full of freckles, Dana had spunk. Most of the time, she paired thin black leggings with a racerback tank top and silver hoop earrings that swung back and forth with each springy step. Dana had ten tattoos, including Paige's name on her left foot and Madison's on the back of her neck. When we first met, Dana showed me one tattoo she was in the painful process of removing: her ex-husband's initials around her ring finger.

A quick-witted and frank conversationalist, Dana paired her opinions with open-mindedness. She had deep convictions, yet that never dampened her curiosity about other viewpoints. Aspects of my life — this research, for instance — seemed strange to her, but she always praised me for doing what made me happy.

Like Nyah, Dana was resilient and optimistic. She was also no stranger to feeling lonely, although she generally didn't feel alone. Her family's support, Dana liked to tell me, was what allowed her to financially and emotionally weather the challenges she had faced over the years: her biological father's alcoholism, her ex-husband's drug addiction and emotional abuse, a tumultuous divorce, and, most recently, her own battle with breast cancer.

At forty years old, Dana had already overcome a lot. When Dana was a baby, her mother left her father — a physically abusive drug addict and alcoholic — and quickly remarried. At fifteen, Dana dropped out of high school and moved out of her mother and stepfather's place and in with her boyfriend. While Dana eventually dumped that boyfriend and went on to earn her GED, the experience taught her the value of independence and grit. At twenty-four, Dana met a man named Justin.

"We fell in love, whatever," Dana said with a laugh as she replayed their romance for me. A year later, Dana gave birth to Madison. Six weeks after that, Justin split, leaving Dana alone to care for their newborn. In the end, Justin gave Madison little else beyond life.

Without child support or a job, Dana moved back in with her mom, Debra. Debra was a wiry, fiercely loyal woman with an eyebrow ring and inability to suffer fools. Debra supported Dana the first year of Madison's life while Dana put herself through medical-assistant school and then secured her first job at a pediatric clinic.

When Madison was four years old, Dana fell in love again. His name was Chris and he was tall with coarse brown hair and a diamond stud in each ear. Chris was ready to commit. A year later, the two got married. Two years after that, Paige was born. Dana thought she had found her happy ending: a loving marriage and a family of four. But Dana soon saw her mother's history repeating itself in her own life. Chris started drinking frequently and dealing and using drugs. Dana intervened, telling him he had to get his act together. On her salary, she put him through rehab, after which his substance use seemed to subside. But when it flared up again two years later, it was accompanied by extreme verbal and psychological abuse.

On Paige's fourth birthday, Dana decided to cut her losses: she filed for divorce and issued a restraining order against Chris. Two months later, she discovered she had breast cancer. The next year was spent in a haze, cycling between courtrooms and chemotherapy.

"I'm a push-go-shove kind of person," Dana said, recounting the most challenging year of her life. "So I pushed and shoved my way through it." Dana devoted whatever energy she had to shielding her girls from the effects of both traumas. Looking back, she was proudest of the fact that nothing changed for Madison and Paige during that year.

"My girls never saw me cry." Dana smiled, tucking a flyaway strand of brown hair behind her ear. "I either cried in the shower or in bed."

Dana survived both the divorce and cancer, successes that she in part attributed to her parents' support. Through it all, Debra had watched both girls. Dana's father, who was now clean, had helped her financially. And her kids—well, her kids were what had kept her going. They were her entire world, her single greatest source of joy.

Dynamic and curious, Madison and Paige endeared themselves to me the first time we met. Madison, who had long dark brown hair, wide eyes, and a cheerleader's physique, had struggled over the years with attention deficit hyperactivity disorder and anxiety, but she had an electricity that could light up the darkest room. With light brown hair, a contagious gap-toothed smile, and boundless energy, Madison's younger sister, Paige, was notoriously affectionate, often snuggling with her mom in bed and meeting me at the front door with a bear hug. The rest of the time, Paige was cracking jokes, impersonating her favorite cartoon characters, or somersaulting across the living room.

Dana was a devoted mother, adaptive to her girls' evolving needs and interests. And whatever time she didn't spend with her kids, she spent trying to support them. Whether that meant working around the clock or calling various camps and sports leagues to inquire about youth scholarships, Dana strove tirelessly to grant her daughters their dreams. For Paige, that meant getting to practice gymnastics and softball. For Madison, it was cheerleading and church camp. What Dana didn't want was for them to have less than meaningful childhoods just because they weren't growing up rich. She wouldn't let them be shortchanged just because she was a single mom.

"I'm their mom and their dad, basically," Dana informed me one afternoon as she poured in the powdered cheese for Paige's mac-and-cheese dinner. She also told me that she had no intention of remarrying. "I refuse for my kids to feel like I'm picking a man over them," Dana explained, stirring the cheese and pasta. "I'm trying to break the cycle."

Part of breaking the cycle involved shielding her daughters from negative influences. Dana, for her part, had resolved to stay clean: no tobacco, no drugs, not even prescription narcotics. "After my double mastectomy and reconstruction," she told me, "I took meds for three days and that was it." When she had her ovaries and fallopian tubes removed, Dana didn't pop one pill. Once a month, she treated herself to a cocktail with her girlfriends. That was the extent of her drinking.

Financially, Dana was close to making ends meet. Her full-time job as a medical assistant with benefits gave her some degree of financial stability and health care for her and her daughters. Even though she was still paying off thousands in credit card debt, didn't receive any child support, and had never opened a savings account, Dana felt that she was managing. Each month, she brought home a little over four thousand dollars. That, coupled with three hundred dollars a month from her dad and his willingness to cover her car payments and half of Madison's cheerleading costs, helped. But Dana's income went fast. Half of her monthly paycheck, about two thousand dollars, she put toward rent and utilities. The rest was divided among cell phone bills, cable bills, gas, trash pickup, and the girls' activities and after-school care. Dana and her brother also paid Debra's rent and cell phone bills. Once a month, Dana treated herself to a manicure.

"People always tell me you have to make your own time." Dana laughed, looking down at her newly polished nails. "But I don't know. Maybe when the girls are all grown."

The Ortegas

"We're a busy family," Renata Ortega told me the first time we met. It was a crisp October morning, and we were standing in the kitchen of the three-bedroom house that Renata and her husband, José, had bought in 2009 for just over $400,000. The Ortegas lived in a middle-class neighborhood lined with single-family homes belonging to Latinx, white, and Asian families. Renata's kids—fourteen-year-old Amalia and twelve-year-old Nico—were on fall break, and Renata was preparing their breakfast. After sautéing two sausage links in a frying pan, she poured in four whisked eggs to make an omelet. When the omelet was ready, she divided it onto two plates and added a handful of oven-baked crinkle-cut fries to each. "Nico! Amalia! Breakfast is ready!" she called to the kids as she carried their plates into the dining room.

Renata, with her wide brown eyes and thick black hair tied in a neat ponytail, had a welcoming, measured demeanor. Warm and patient, Renata could calm even the most frayed of nerves. That morning, she wore gray pin-striped trousers and a black V-neck shirt featuring the logo of the bank where she worked as a business manager.

Renata was a fourth-generation Mexican-American. Her husband, José, was third-generation. Both were born and raised in the Bay Area, Renata as a self-identified latchkey kid. Her father, a Vietnam veteran, became an engineer, and her mother held jobs as a telephone operator, teacher's aide, and small-business owner. Together, Renata's parents worked hard to open doors for their kids. While Renata's brothers spent much of their time on the soccer field, Renata's passion was dance. It was a love she carried through her high-school and college years, performing on the sidelines for sports teams and in a major dance company.

Upon graduating from San Francisco State University, Renata began her career in commercial banking. A few years later, a friend set her up with José, a tall man with gelled black hair and a soft smile who was nine years her senior. José didn't have Renata's college degree, but he was both a successful musician and a salesman for technology products. After a couple of years of dating, the two got married and had Amalia. Renata had always wanted a family of four, and two years after Amalia was born, she got her wish when she gave birth to a son, Gabriel. But at just three months old, soon after Renata returned to work, Gabriel passed away from sudden infant death syndrome.

The tragic loss of their son forever changed Renata and José. "You cannot imagine what it's like to go through something like that," Renata told me. The loss took a toll on them as individuals and as partners. But in that utter darkness, Renata and José uncovered something new: their faith. Turning to God and the church, they found hope and purpose in Christianity.

"Church became the platform for us to heal, pick up the pieces, and rebuild our lives," Renata said, smiling. Their faith also became a centerpiece of their family life, helping them "beat the odds." Most marriages, Renata knew, didn't survive the loss of a child.

In the end, their son Nico's arrival gave Renata the family of four she'd always longed for. That family became everything to her. As a mom, Renata was a devoted Energizer Bunny and an eternal optimist. The kids and their interests and activities kept her and José very busy, which was how they liked it. One evening as we sat on the couch watching TV, Renata told me about her recent career transition. After two decades working at one bank, five years ago she moved to a different bank, Metropolitan Trust.

"I told Metro that I needed to be able to prioritize my family," she explained. "If my kids need me, then I have to be able to pick them up and tend to them."

Amalia and Nico were easygoing and amiable like their mom. With coarse brown hair woven into two long braids, Amalia had high cheekbones and smiled often. Nico had light brown hair and a calm energy. Both kids were involved in the performing arts, church youth groups, modeling, and commercial acting. Many of the hours I spent at Renata's side were in the passenger seat of her Ford Fusion as she shuttled Amalia and Nico around to their various extracurriculars.

Renata traced her devotion to her kids back to her own childhood. "Growing up," she told me, "we didn't feel poor. But looking back now, I see that we were kinda poor." When Renata was growing up, she knew that her parents worked hard, even scrambling at times to make ends meet. She knew they had outstanding debts on at least a dozen credit cards. She also recalled a brief period when they were both out of work. Money was so tight then that in order to pay their mortgage, they had to cash in the savings bonds they'd bought her and her two brothers.

But whatever financial hardships her parents endured, they made sure Renata never suffered the effects. They sacrificed to deliver Renata a vibrant childhood packed with dance recitals and competitions. They never skimped on anything for their daughter's dancing, whether that meant covering the hotels for overnight competitions or buying the glitteriest outfit to help Renata shine onstage. Reflecting on everything her parents had done for her, Renata was clear about one thing. She wanted to provide the same for her own children.

"I feel that we are doing that for our kids now," Renata told me, smiling. Compared to her parents, Renata believed, she and José were in a more comfortable position to offer their kids active, fulfilling childhoods. She also felt that, health-wise, they were prepared to do this. Renata, who was in her mid-forties, was mindful of her family history of high blood pressure and diabetes. But apart from her marginally high cholesterol and José's high blood pressure, they were in good shape.

Renata wished they made more money, but she appreciated what they had. Together, Renata and José brought in around $175,000 a year. They had a mortgage, but they also had savings and retirement accounts. Their kids were enrolled in good public schools, and once a year they took a family vacation.

"At least we own our home!" Renata said. This was indeed a remarkable thing in an area with a median home price of $928,000. Still, Renata told me, she sometimes worried. "We still feel like we're living paycheck to paycheck."

The Cains

I first met Julie Cain in the foyer of the two-story, four-bedroom house she shared with her husband, Zach, and their two kids, thirteen-year-old Jane and seventeen-year-old Evan. Just a fifteen-minute drive from the Ortegas, the Cains lived on a quiet cul-de-sac in a largely white, upper-middle-class residential neighborhood. That day, their home was decorated in anticipation of Halloween in two weeks. Outside, pumpkins of assorted shapes and sizes lined the front steps. Inside, kitchen countertops and the fireplace mantel were covered with pumpkin-, witch-, and ghost-themed decorations.

When I rang the doorbell that first afternoon, I heard Max, the Cains' border collie, scurry across the living room to greet me, his toenails tapping on the hardwood floors. Julie followed, calling his name to quiet his barking. Julie, who was in her mid-forties, had short, straight, straw-blond hair that she wore in a layered bob. Warm and affable, Julie had a bellowing laugh that echoed off the kitchen tiles and an unmistakably Midwestern hospitality. She also carried the remnants of a Midwestern twang even though it had been decades since she'd called the middle of the country home.

Julie had a casual, polished style. She was often sporting a cardigan with skinny jeans, athleisure-style leggings and tank tops, or, on a summer afternoon, a T-shirt with khaki shorts. Her oversize Longchamp tote and reusable water bottle accompanied her wherever she went, the latter filled with bubbly water from her SodaStream machine. While Julie's demeanor communicated a traditional approach to life, she was, deep down, a free spirit. One afternoon, as the two of us sat outside the Cains' temple at a picnic table while Jane was inside preparing with the rabbi for her bat mitzvah, Julie pulled up her pant leg. "I got a tattoo," she said, smiling, her voice filled with mischievous delight. It had hurt, and Zach had jokingly called it a tramp stamp. But Julie loved it, and she especially enjoyed that she and her girlfriends had all visited the tattoo parlor together. "It was soccer-mom Saturday at that tattoo parlor," she said with a chuckle, pulling the pant leg back down.

With her kids, Julie was loving and spirited. She had been a stay-at-home mom for the past seventeen years, and Evan and Jane were her whole world. For that, she felt truly lucky, mentioning more than once how fortunate she had been to be able to stay home with them since the day they were born.

Julie had called the Bay Area home for the past fifteen years, but she was used to moving around. While she was growing up, her father's jobs in retail and insurance had taken the family all over the country. When Julie was a high-school sophomore, her parents announced that they were moving to Alabama. "That was probably the most traumatic part of my childhood," Julie said. "Having to move my junior year." Other than that, Julie had fond memories from her youth, including her parents' happy marriage. Her mother, who worked part-time as a secretary, was always home after school to care for Julie and her younger sister.

"Nothing extraordinary or extreme happened in my childhood." Julie smiled.

For college, Julie headed east to Georgia to study communications. At graduation, she met Zach, a California-born lawyer who had just passed the bar and was clerking for a judge. After two years of dating, they had a country-club wedding. Zach's job in corporate law sent them briefly to Mississippi and then to Kentucky, where Evan was born. Two years later, they headed to California, where they welcomed Jane. The Cains moved around the Bay Area for a while, renting houses before finally purchasing their current home in 2008 for just under a million dollars.

Broad-shouldered with slicked-back gray hair and a goatee, Zach was an extrovert with a cutting sarcasm. Most of the time I spent with the Cains, Zach wasn't home. He was generally at the office, putting in long hours as in-house counsel for a global technology company. Other times, he was at the gym or entertaining clients at business dinners. Jane and Evan were chatty and gregarious. Jane had long, curly red hair, a bubbly demeanor, and her dad's disarming sense of humor. An avid dancer and volleyball player, Jane was navigating eighth grade while touring private high schools for the next year. Evan, who was tall with shiny brown hair and a wide smile, exuded a casual warmth that could set a room at ease. He had a mild case of senioritis and devoted most of his after-school hours to theater. He would soon be graduating from prep school and heading off to college at the University of Southern California in Los Angeles.

In anticipation of becoming an empty nester, Julie was considering going back to work part-time. But she struggled to figure out what she might excel at after so many years out of the workforce. She updated her LinkedIn profile and sent her résumé around while keeping busy. Julie spent most afternoons and evenings behind the wheel of her Mercedes SUV shuttling Jane to and from extracurricular activities. Beyond that, there were exercise classes, lunches with friends, and errands to run. Julie also served on the boards of her Jewish temple and a local mother-daughter charity organization.

While Julie had an active social life, I sensed that some of the loneliness I'd felt in Nyah, Dana, and Renata lived in her as well. It lived in a lot of the moms I met. I sometimes wondered if that was a reason they let me hang around. *Did they enjoy the company?* I wondered. One evening, Julie and I sat at the kitchen counter eating homemade pizza. Evan and Jane were gone, and Zach was swinging by the gym after a long day at work. "At least you're here to spend time with me!" she joked. But I knew that behind that laugh lay a kernel of truth.

Julie and Zach were largely in good health. While Julie thought Zach could afford to lose some weight, she left that largely to him to manage. With Jane, however, she and Zach both intervened when they felt their daughter was struggling with her weight. Consulting with their pediatrician and hiring a nutritionist and a therapist, they had tried over the past couple of years to help Jane make different dietary choices. "It's been a huge topic

of discussion in our family," Julie said with a sigh late one afternoon as the two of us chopped tomatoes at the kitchen counter.

Financially, the Cains were worlds apart from the Bakers,
Williamses, and Ortegas. Each year, Zach brought home a little
under half a million dollars. The Cains owned a home now
worth almost four times that. They were still paying the mortgage but were otherwise debt-free. Evan's yearly high-school
tuition ran around twenty thousand dollars, and Jane's would
soon run a similar amount. That fall, the Cains were paying for
Evan's college tours and college applications. The kids' extracurriculars also broke into the thousands. During my time with
the Cains, they took spontaneous cross-country trips to visit
family, purchased front-row tickets to concerts, and planned a
family cruise.

Still, even with their financial cushion, the Cains saw the
Bay Area as too expensive for them long term. "We have a good
life here," Julie told me one afternoon as we drove home from
the dry cleaner's. "But it's still competitive and expensive, so I
don't think it's a good place to retire."

Julie, Renata, Dana, and Nyah came from divergent backgrounds and parented their kids with wildly different resources.
At first glance, it might have seemed as though they didn't share
much beyond motherhood. But that one commonality, in many
ways, united them more poignantly than all their differences
could divide them. Each of these moms felt an aching love for
her children. Each had a fierce instinct to protect them. Each
held a deeply rooted desire to see her kids grow into healthy and
happy adults. These sentiments underpinned how all four moms
approached their kids' diets. But as I soon came to learn, the
vastly different resources moms had at their disposal to act on
these feelings translated into vastly different approaches to
nourishing the ones they loved.

CHAPTER 3

Feeding Kids

When Nyah Baker was a child, her aunt used to sauté fresh spinach leaves with a generous heap of butter and minced garlic. From their bedroom down the hall, Nyah and her sisters could hear the handfuls of leafy greens hit the sizzling frying pan in the kitchen. Moments later, a distinctly earthy smell would waft through the house, and they would start to gag.

"Me and my sisters," Nyah recalled, laughing. "We used to go, 'Ew, this stinks!'" Despising its bitter taste and slimy texture, they would beg their aunt not to make spinach for dinner. When they found it on their plates, the protests would begin. But Nyah's aunt had zero tolerance for her nieces' gripes. Spinach was part of what was for dinner, and they weren't getting any of their favorite dishes — potato salad, fried chicken, pork chops — until they got down at least one helping of the soggy vegetable. Nyah would hold her nose and force down bite after bite, wincing as she swallowed. For encouragement, Nyah's aunt would remind Nyah of the cartoon character Popeye, whose spinach-rich diet was responsible for his bulging biceps. "You want to be strong like that man!" her aunt would chime in over the sound of Nyah's pained gulps. While Nyah resented her aunt at the time, that resentment blossomed into gratitude over the years.

"Now," Nyah said with a grin, "I love spinach!"

To get her own daughters to try the greens she once loathed, Nyah called on her aunt's cartoon character from thirty years ago. "I tell them about Popeye too." Nyah laughed. "And they buy it. They thinkin', *I'ma be strong!*" Now Mariah and Natasha loved greens of all kinds. They would gobble up spinach, collard greens, and chard, all of which were packed with vitamins and nutrients that Nyah knew were healthy and good for their development.

Spinach was just one nutritious food Nyah wanted her girls to eat. Plenty of other fruits, vegetables, and meats made good choices in her book. A nutritious diet was important because it would make her daughters strong and healthy, Nyah told me. It would also help them sidestep challenges Nyah had faced because of her health, including high blood pressure and diabetes. Nyah wanted Mariah and Natasha to get the nutrition they needed to thrive, be active, and live long and fulfilling lives.

Dana Williams, Renata Ortega, and Julie Cain all felt the same way. So did most moms I met. Dana's experiences working in the medical field as well as her recent battle with breast cancer had underscored for her the profound importance of a healthy diet. Dana didn't want her daughters drinking soda or eating dessert before dinner. She hoped they'd never become part of the increasingly "sick society" she saw all around her.

"They should know they have to eat healthy," Dana said. "We only have one body."

Renata similarly told me that it was critical for her kids to make healthy choices, eat fruits and vegetables, and learn how to eat the right portions for their hunger and bodies. "We do try to eat healthy," she told me one morning as we sat side by side at her dining-room table drinking water. When Renata took Amalia and Nico grocery shopping, she taught them how to make those healthy choices. She told them to choose whole wheat over white bread and advised them to pick fruits that were ripe and that were easy to take to school.

Julie also wanted her kids to eat nutritiously so they wouldn't face debilitating health conditions. Sitting down to a healthy meal each night, Julie told me, was fundamental to kids' health and well-being. Julie considered herself fortunate to live in a time when there was so much knowledge about how to eat well. "I know more today than I knew ten years ago," she said, "and I can just imagine what my kids are gonna know in ten years!"

Moms up and down the income spectrum resoundingly echoed these four women. If anything was clear to me, it was this: Most moms cared deeply about their kids' diets and health. During our conversations, only a handful didn't raise the importance of a healthy diet for their kids; the vast majority connected the dots between kids' diets and their current and future health. Moms articulated their desire for their children to eat healthy in order to *be* healthy. They told me that healthy food was an investment in their kids' well-being, that it was medicine, and that it was key to living a long, healthy life. As one mom put it, "Your health is gonna depend on what you put into your body. Period."

I was similarly struck by the fact that moms were largely aligned on what they meant by *healthy*. There was more consensus than disagreement. Vegetables, fruits, whole grains, fish, and lean meats—these were what most deemed nutritious choices. Many also talked about the importance of eating organic, fresh, homemade, or whole foods. The virtues of drinking water were regularly extolled. In contrast, soda, candy, chips, fried and fast foods, and foods high in fat, salt, or sugar—moms agreed that these were less than ideal and unhealthy choices. Sugar was widely condemned, with moms underscoring its negative consequences for their kids' teeth and weight, its addictive properties, and the sneaky inclusion of it in so many of the most tempting foods.[1]

Of course, there were also differences in how moms defined *healthy*. Some thought foods higher in protein—such as meat—were healthier; others saw more plant-based diets as equally or more nutritious. Some viewed starchy foods like bread and cereal as healthy choices; others wrote those off as empty calories. Some believed there was a place for fruit juice in their kids' diets; others saw such drinks as an inadequate and unhealthy substitute for fresh fruit. Still, even with these differences, I was overwhelmed by the degree to which moms' ideas about healthy eating and the value they placed on it converged.[2]

When it came to how families actually ate, there were also striking similarities. Most families I met shopped primarily at supermarkets. Most fridges had some amount of fresh food, like fruits, vegetables, raw meat, bread, and dairy. Families' freezers were packed with frozen vegetables, frozen pizzas, and party appetizers. Dana always had pizza rolls, Nyah chicken drumsticks, Renata bagel bites, and Julie ice cream.

Most cabinets were lined with packaged and processed foods. In Renata's pantry, I found jasmine rice and canned tomatoes as well as Ritz crackers, fruit cups, Capri Sun pouches, and cans of Spam. Julie's pantry was filled with the latest Trader Joe's nonperishable creations, like pumpkin-flavored cereal, cookies, pastas, popcorn, and pretzels. One October morning, I saw Julie put together a breakfast of pumpkin pancakes with pumpkin butter and pumpkin-spice maple syrup alongside a cup of pumpkin-spice coffee. Nyah's cabinets were overflowing with canned vegetables, beans, soups, and sauces, plus bags of chips and nuts. Dana's included rows of boxed mac and cheese, Froot Loops, Oreos, and Kool-Aid.

Given the powerful reach of the food and beverage industry into families' lives, the abundance of less nutritious, processed foods in families' homes didn't surprise me. All year round, Big Food and Big Beverage use powerful advertising and marketing to regularly bombard Americans with images of these items. In 2017, food companies spent eleven billion dollars on television ads, 80 percent of which were for their unhealthiest offerings, including soda, fast food, candy, and snacks.[3] These foods are also inexpensive and engineered to be delicious. When you pair those qualities with the fact that these foods are virtually everywhere, it's easy to see how they become appealing choices for busy moms and families.

During my time with families, I saw how the food industry pushed the foods mothers, fathers, and children most often encountered in daily life. On their daily commutes to work and school, billboard advertisements for Pizza Hut and radio ads for Lay's grabbed their attention. During their evenings in front of the television, Jack in the Box commercials and Pepsi product placements caught their eyes. These foods also appeared as advertisements on Instagram and Twitter feeds and embedded in news articles and clothing sites. At the supermarket, two-for-one deals on Hamburger Helper and Chex cereal pulled the mothers I met away from full-priced heads of broccoli and cartons of eggs. As I weaved through grocery aisles at the sides of these moms, I noted how fresh foods formed a thin outer ring around the store while processed products made up the bulk of the middle.[4] Processed foods also beckoned to families from checkout lanes in every Nordstrom Rack and Bed, Bath, and Beyond. Even Office Depot had a full aisle packed with chips, soda, and candy alongside other aisles of printer paper, whiteboards, and writing utensils. When families went out to eat, persuasive marketing tactics—supersizing, meal deals, and buy-one-get-one-free offers—tempted them to consume more nutritionally dubious foods.

Together, these tactics encouraged families to put their dollars toward ever-present and appetizing but less nutritious foods.[5] These tactics are also a major reason why the American food environment—that is, the physical and social surroundings shaping our diets—is generally considered, at best, difficult to navigate and, at worst, toxic. The fact is that the overwhelming abundance of food promotions and "deals" makes it much easier, financially, physically, and psychologically, for Americans to eat less healthy foods.[6] The result was that not one of the four families I spent time with escaped food corporations' long reach.

On weekdays, most families ate at home. Nyah and Julie cooked almost every day, Dana and Renata a few days each week. Some moms re-created at least a couple of dishes from their childhoods, and every family had a few family favorites on steady rotation. Dishes like pasta, tacos, and pizza graced many tables.

I ate garlic bread independently with Nyah, Dana, Renata, and Julie. These meals often had a joyful element to them. For most families, food was central to holidays and celebrations. It could also be fun and delicious. Dana and her kids loved having breakfast for dinner. Dana would whip up instant pancakes while the girls set the table with unsalted butter and real maple syrup. Nyah and Marcus enjoyed spending weekend afternoons making okra, mac and cheese, and pork chops the mouthwatering way Nyah's grandmother had taught her to twenty years ago.

Most families also ate food from outside the home, sometimes during the week and even more commonly on weekends. For some, that meant frequenting restaurants. For others, it meant cruising through the drive-through, ordering takeout, joining family potlucks, or picking up a pizza during a run to Costco. Try as they might to resist, almost every single family I met at least occasionally indulged in the kinds of American classics featured in fast-food advertisements: a juicy burger, chicken wings, French fries, or onion rings.

And yet, despite the similarities that bound families across society, their diets diverged in important ways.

First, although most families shopped primarily in supermarkets, they chose different ones. Wealthier families frequented pricier supermarkets like Whole Foods, Safeway, and Trader Joe's; lower-income families occasionally popped into these stores but shopped more regularly at places like Lucky's, Walmart, Target, and discount grocers like FoodMaxx or dollar stores. Some lower-income families received food from food banks, although many did so only under what they deemed "extreme" circumstances; going to the food bank wasn't something families did casually. In the supermarket, wealthier families often purchased organic foods; most, if not all, of their fruits and vegetables were organic. Lower-income families bought conventional fruits and vegetables. They purchased organic foods only rarely—for instance, when they were heavily discounted.

Wealthier families also tended to keep more fresh produce around than low-income families, who had a larger share of more processed, nonperishable products.

Families also talked about food in different ways. While moms across income levels shared similar dietary wishes for their kids, wealthier moms mentioned far more food-related rules at home. These moms discussed—often at great length—restrictions they had placed on their children's diets. They also described having more dietary "teaching moments" and instructional conversations with kids. Lower-income moms, however, mentioned far fewer rules and restrictions around food with their kids. They did not have the same kinds of "teaching moments" or conversations about dietary health.[7] As similar as families seemed in some ways, the deeper I dug, the more clearly I saw how dramatically their dietary habits and beliefs diverged.

What accounted for these dietary differences across families?

This was the question that many public health scholars proposed we already knew the answer to—dietary differences, I'd read, were driven by differences in people's access to healthy food. Fix food access, I'd been told, and you'll close the dietary gap.

To many of us, the food-access argument is better and more widely known by its buzzword: *food deserts*. A food desert, according to the USDA, is a low-income census tract where at least a third of the population lives more than one mile from a supermarket in an urban area and more than ten miles from one in a rural area. While the USDA definition requires a neighborhood to be low income to be considered a food desert, people often use the term to refer to any neighborhood where it's hard to find fresh fruits and vegetables—for instance, neighborhoods without any affordable (or any) supermarkets. Lower-income neighborhoods more often fit this colloquial understanding of what constitutes a food desert; while a fourth of all zip codes in the United States lack a supermarket, that number doubles for zip codes with a median income below $25,000, and slightly over half of those very-low-income areas have no supermarket at all.

The more I read about food access, the more I wondered where the term had come from and why it had become so widely accepted as *the* driving force behind nutritional inequality.

In the United States, the concept of food access was popularized quickly and dramatically by First Lady Michelle Obama's Let's Move! campaign to end childhood obesity. The campaign was a watershed period in the American healthy-eating movement—it raised widespread awareness about food and health as issues of social justice and made swift strides to prevent and treat childhood obesity.

Some of these strides were political; others were symbolic. Michelle Obama launched the first-ever Task Force on Childhood Obesity, which created a national action plan to mobilize public and private sectors and engage communities to improve kids' health. The opening of the White House vegetable garden made a powerful statement about dietary health. On the policy front, the Healthy, Hunger-Free Kids Act of 2010 offered a momentous step toward improving school food; it updated school-meal nutrition standards for the first time in fifteen years and increased funding for the first time in thirty years. The act provided $4.5 billion in new federal funding for school-meal and child-nutrition programs over a decade, leading American public schools to start offering healthier meals and snacks to over fifty million kids.[8] The First Lady also recognized the powerful, pernicious reach of the food industry and worked to limit students' exposure to unhealthy food marketing. While many of the improvements to school food made during the Obama administration were ultimately rolled back under President Trump between 2016 and 2020, the newfound awareness and visibility of these issues could not be undone.

The Let's Move! campaign also popularized the idea that childhood obesity stemmed in part from inadequate geographic food access. It was an idea with immediate, broad resonance and an accessible avenue for talking about inequalities in nutrition and health. Michelle Obama made eliminating food deserts a central element of her broader campaign, the underlying assumption being that poor children (many of whom were children of color) were obese because their families did not have access to healthy foods. By increasing families' and neighborhoods' access to healthy food, kids' nutrition would improve. Over time, obesity rates would fall. The argument had wide appeal because it offered a straightforward, actionable solution. It also helpfully shifted the blame away from individuals and families, instead highlighting structural constraints and suggesting that the deck was stacked against them. If access was the problem, then the fix was clear: open supermarkets in low-income communities.

Over the next decade, Herculean national, state, and local policy efforts followed to increase low-income communities' access to healthy food. By 2010, the USDA had quantified and mapped food deserts across the country, created an online food-desert locator, and instituted National Food Desert Awareness Month. Federal and state programs provided loans, grants, and tax credits to stimulate supermarket development and encourage retailers to offer healthy foods in food deserts. The federal government launched the Healthy Food Financing Initiative to support retailers running supermarkets in low-income areas, providing $400 million for the program and $250 million in tax credits. Overall, the coordinated, collaborative effort to invest in underserved communities and bring healthy food into food deserts was widely successful.

But if the goal of those efforts was to improve families' diet quality and reduce childhood obesity, the initiatives were surprisingly disappointing. Over the years, a growing number of studies have assessed the impact of opening supermarkets in food deserts. While research has shown that supermarket openings increase residents' perceptions that they have access to healthy food, these openings have little to no effect on residents' diets and physical health. Most notably, two major studies in

Philadelphia and New York City found new supermarkets brought no significant change to food-desert residents' diets.[9] Other studies have echoed these findings, underscoring a disappointing reality: improving food access does little to improve poor communities' diet quality. Food access, it turns out, doesn't explain much of the nutritional inequality in the United States.[10]

Geographic access to healthy food seemed to play a negligible role in the diets of the seventy-five families I met. Because I knew where every family lived, I could map families' distance from supermarkets and use the USDA's online food-desert tracker to see whether they lived in a food desert or an area with low food access. Together, my own maps and the federal tracker revealed to me that most families had high geographic access to healthy food. None resided in food deserts, and almost all lived within two miles of a supermarket.

I seriously considered whether my measure of food access was leading me astray. While it was capturing families' proximity to supermarkets, perhaps what mattered more than objective geographic access to food was subjective access. Did families *feel* like they could get ahold of the food they wanted and needed? Did they feel physically cut off from it? Maybe the supermarkets near families were too expensive, too limited, or too alienating. Maybe the lines were too long or the produce underripe.

As I pored over the transcripts of my conversations with families, it became clear to me that families' subjective perceptions of food access matched their objective realities. To my enormous surprise, families simply didn't see geographic access as an issue. Almost every mom said she had access to an affordable supermarket nearby. In fact, I found that in the largely suburban context of the Bay Area, the vast majority of families owned cars that they could use to drive to the supermarket. The two families that didn't have a car both lived within half a mile of a grocery store. In the end, while moms told me, at great length, about all kinds of challenges and constraints when it came to feeding their families, physically accessing the food they wanted just wasn't one of them.[11] Differences in families' geographic access to healthy food didn't explain their different diets.

While I didn't know it back in 2014, emerging research since has helped explain why food deserts and geographic food access don't matter as much as we once thought. National statistics on car use mirror what I saw among my families: the vast majority of U.S. households today (over 90 percent) have access to a car. And a 2019 study using real consumer data found that, like the parents I met, most people are also actually quite willing to travel for their groceries. In fact, the average American travels 5.2 miles to grocery shop, and 90 percent of shopping trips in the country are made by car. It turns out that people are quite okay with traveling longer distances to buy food and are less geographically constrained than formerly thought. Because of that, when a new supermarket is set up in a neighborhood, most residents simply shift from shopping at a more distant supermarket—not a gas station or bodega—to the closer one. Ultimately, the study's authors estimated that just 10 percent of socioeconomic diet disparities in the United States can be traced to differences in access to healthy food. That leaves the other *90 percent* of the nutritional gap unaccounted for.[12]

Of course there is more to food access than geography. Financial access to food, healthy food in particular, matters too. Among the families I met, financial access offered a more promising explanation for dietary differences than geographic access. In the United States, lower-income families spend less on food than higher-income ones do—$3,767 a year, compared to $12,340 a year for the wealthiest households. Poorer families also devote a greater proportion of their household income to food—33 percent of their earnings go to food, compared to wealthier households' 9 percent.[13]

Many Americans also simply don't have enough money to buy food. This is best evidenced by the fact that in 2018, forty million Americans participated each month in the federal government's Supplemental Nutrition Assistance Program, also known as

SNAP.[14] SNAP provides financial support for food for low-income Americans—two-thirds of whom are families with children. SNAP's monthly stipends rarely provide families with enough funds to buy nutritious meals for an entire month. This is in part because the program was designed to be supplemental and to *assist* families, not to guarantee them sufficient amounts of healthy food. Its modest benefits—averaging less than just $1.40 per person per meal—are hardly enough to cover families' monthly food costs.[15]

The allotments also inadequately account for the reality that healthier food generally costs more than unhealthier food.[16] Calorie for calorie, more nutritious staples like lean meats, fish, fruits, and vegetables are more expensive than less nutritious foods higher in refined grains and added sugar. It's true that a tomato can be cheaper than a bag of chips and that a head of cauliflower sometimes costs less than chicken nuggets. But these calculations take neither calories nor quantities into account. For families living hand to mouth, trying to maximize overall caloric intake can mean purchasing more food for less money. This incentivizes families to make their dollars stretch by purchasing cheaper, unhealthier foods.

The families I met spent vastly different amounts on food each month, from less than $200 to over $1,000. Nyah, Dana, Renata, and Julie illustrated this variation, spending around $300, $360, $450, and $900 each month on food, respectively.[17] Their spending patterns also echoed national data showing that higher-income families spend more on food overall, but lower-income families spend a greater share of their income on it. While Julie and Renata each spent more overall on food than Nyah and Dana, Nyah and Dana put a comparatively larger chunk of their earnings toward it.

Nyah, like many low-income moms I met, depended on safety-net benefits to feed her family. Many families below the poverty line, like hers, used SNAP, and some low-income pregnant moms or those with young children also depended on Women, Infants, and Children (WIC) benefits. Undocumented parents, who were almost always low-income, were not eligible for SNAP but were at times able to access WIC benefits.[18]

Marcus's SNAP funds kept Nyah and the girls fed each month. Technically, Nyah explained to me once, Marcus was homeless. He registered his blue van rather than Nyah's house as his residence. Doing so made him a member of a separate household, which entitled him to his own separate public benefits. Each month, Marcus received $194 in SNAP funds to buy food.[19] When those funds arrived on the first of the month, Nyah would spend them immediately at a discount grocer. Wandering the aisles, she would fill the shopping cart to the brim with foods to last her family until the first of the next month. She bought greens like spinach to cook that week, but almost everything else that made it into the cart was nonperishable, since it had to last thirty days without rotting. As backup, Nyah kept a freezer in the garage full of frozen meat and her cupboards stocked with canned corn, beans, and ravioli. Most months, Nyah supplemented Marcus's benefits with one hundred dollars of her daughters' SSI stipends.[20] She used some of that money on groceries, and the rest went to takeout food and beer, both of which were unallowable purchases under SNAP. Sometimes, this was enough to carry her family through the month.

Other times, it wasn't.

Nyah, like roughly half of all households participating in SNAP and a third of single mothers in the United States, was food-insecure. Being food-insecure meant that she had unreliable access to a sufficient amount of affordable, nutritious food. Food insecurity in the United States affects more than thirty-five million people and about two-thirds of households below the poverty line. In 2019, one in nine Americans lacked enough food.[21] In 2020, the economic hardship brought on by the coronavirus pandemic significantly worsened the problem; food insecurity rates in the U.S. doubled, affecting around one in five households. What's more, the rate for families with children tripled; just short of one in three families with kids experienced food insecurity that year.[22]

Food insecurity is associated with a less healthy diet for a number of reasons. First, uncertain and insufficient access to enough food incentivizes people to purchase higher quantities of cheaper and often less nutritious food to ensure they will get enough calories. Indeed, food-insecure individuals are more likely to consume salty snacks, sugar-sweetened beverages, and red or processed meat.[23] For the same reason, food insecurity also financially incentivizes families to purchase more energy-dense, satiating foods, such as full-fat dairy products, nuts, seeds, and legumes. While many of these foods are nutritious, they may also be high in fat, sodium, and calories. Finally, food insecurity subjects people to repeated periods of food restriction or deprivation, making them more likely to overeat when food becomes available. This feast-or-famine cycle is exactly how both hunger and obesity can coexist in the same communities and even in the same people.[24]

Nyah's resourcefulness is what allowed her to make the foods she bought last. But if things got really tight, she would rely on her sister Dominique or the local food pantry to make ends meet. Nyah once told me that part of surviving as a mom was "using what I got to get what I want." Then she paused. "As long as I am a woman, I should never be broke, and my kids should always have food to eat."

Nyah was the first to admit that the food her kids ate wasn't as healthy as it could be. She made sure I understood that the day we met. "I'ma keep it real," she told me as we plopped down side by side on her sofa. "I buy a lot of junk food. Snacks like doughnuts, Nutty Buddies, the popcorn, and stuff like that— chips, sodas. We always buy Hot Pockets, corn dogs."

Then she pulled two packages of the chocolate and marshmallow cookies known as Moon Pies from her sweatshirt pocket. "You know," she said as she set them on the sofa arm, "fat-girl snacks."

Compared to Nyah's, Dana's earnings put her in a slightly

better position to feed her family. While Dana had at times received SNAP, she was earning too much to qualify when I met her. Still, Dana kept a pretty tight food budget, spending no more than three hundred dollars a month on groceries, plus another sixty dollars on eating out. A savvy Costco shopper, Dana would stock up on large quantities of her kids' favorite foods: chips, pasta, pesto, cream cheese, and milk. She bought the rest of what she needed at Target, which had less expensive generic versions of brand-name favorites. Purchasing organic was, for financial reasons, not on Dana's radar. I never saw Dana buy vegetables, and I saw her buy fruit only once. Often, I witnessed Dana pile the shopping cart with the processed foods her daughters asked for and then lament the high price of healthier options like grapes and bananas. Dana told me that healthy food was more expensive and that she sometimes didn't have the money to buy what she wanted the girls to eat.

"I was going on a big salad and vegetable kick the last few weeks," she told me one evening as we drove home from the nail salon. "I feel like it is expensive—you buy lettuce, and all those little things are expensive. And then you go to the frozen-food section and why are all these TV dinners one dollar? It's so backwards!" One week, I watched Dana partake in a juice cleanse, purchasing and consuming six bottles of premade juices daily at a cost of just over thirty dollars a day. But most of the time, Dana and her daughters ate leftovers and repurposed meals. Sometimes the girls complained, but Dana explained to them that it wasn't up for debate. "If you think you're too cool for leftovers," she said, laughing, "then I'm sorry!"

Renata also worked to stay within a food budget and be mindful of her purchases. She spent around four hundred fifty dollars each month, two hundred fifty on groceries and the rest on takeout food and dining out. Inside Renata's home, I often saw pizza boxes from Papa John's on the kitchen counter and family-size containers of Panda Express on the top shelf of the fridge. Renata shopped at a variety of places, including a higher-end supermarket and a discount grocer. She often bought generic brands. She was wary of food spoiling and preferred to make two runs to the grocery store during the week rather than risk having to throw away moldy grapes or a stale loaf of bread. She didn't worry about having enough food, but she also didn't feel like she could just buy whatever she wanted without first checking how much it cost. If they had more money, Renata once told me, maybe her eyes wouldn't dart to the price tag so readily. Overall, while Renata felt that healthy food was expensive, she also believed it was within her reach. She had the money to buy the fresh foods that she wanted, especially if she sprang for conventional over organic produce.

At the top of the income spectrum, Julie rarely, if ever, made financially motivated food choices. Julie shopped at a variety of places, including Safeway, Target, and Costco. But her absolute favorite store was Trader Joe's. She bought almost exclusively organic fruits and vegetables. When pressed, neither Julie nor Zach could pinpoint exactly how much they spent on food each month. I noted that lower-income moms could effortlessly share with me their monthly food expenditures while wealthier moms like Julie often struggled to come up with an amount. Julie once told me that they spent "way more than five hundred dollars a month" on groceries, in addition to eating out. Together, Julie and I estimated that her family spent around nine hundred dollars each month on food. While she tried to keep their spending "within a reasonable amount," Julie found it difficult to do that and purchase everything she wanted for her family. One challenge was that she was a self-identified last-minute shopper and, as she said with an eye-roll, a "terrible planner." I often saw Julie make two to four trips to the supermarket in one week, and the Cains usually went out to eat once or twice a week. Both Julie and Zach joked that they wished Julie was a little financially savvier when it came to grocery shopping. "But," Julie said with a sigh, "I'm not a coupon cutter."

———————

So maybe price is what matters most, I thought one morning as I typed families' food budgets into the spreadsheet where I logged information from every family I met. I could clearly see how their finances influenced their diets. And yet, as I mulled that idea over, a confusing conversation I'd recently had with Nyah kept coming to mind.

On a Thursday afternoon, I'd sat on a backless stool at Nyah's laminate kitchen counter watching Nyah and Marcus fry batches of chicken drumsticks coated in garlic powder and flour. As Marcus plunged each drumstick into a tall, steel pot of boiling oil, Nyah flipped the cooked ones onto a paper-towel-lined plate to remove the excess grease.

Nyah caught me eyeing two boxes of cereal atop her fridge. "Those are from the free-food box," she said, motioning to the cartons of wheat-bran flakes and plain O's that had captured my attention. Every couple of months, Nyah collected a free box of food from her local pantry. But it often came filled with items she neither recognized nor knew how best to use. What exactly was she supposed to do with celery, saltines, and canned pears?

"No one actually eats those." Nyah grabbed the box of O's and passed it to me. "Why don't you try them?" she said, chuckling, adding that if I liked them, they were mine. I shook the cardboard to dump some O's into the palm of my hand and tasted a few.

"They're pretty plain," I said, chewing slowly. "But, um, they're okay." I thought they tasted a bit like the cardboard box they'd come from.

"Exactly!" Nyah laughed. "The kids don't like 'em either."

What the girls *did* like were Trix and Cinnamon Toast Crunch, Cookie Crunch and Fruity Pebbles. I smiled as Nyah explained that sometimes she could get the girls to eat these healthier cereals if she let them mix a spoonful of sugar into the milk. "It's not good," she said, shrugging. "But I can't blame them!"

Healthier food in Nyah's home is going to waste, I scribbled in my notebook, my hand accidentally smearing the ink as I wrote.

Nyah doesn't just buy the sugary cereals because they're cheap. She buys them because her kids like them. They eat them.

Nyah told me that last year, she had gone on a health kick. For weeks, she'd bought only healthy food: Fruits and vegetables, lean meats, and low-fat dairy. No junk food. Nothing processed.

"Was that expensive?" I asked her, downing another handful of O's. Even though they were flavorless and dried my mouth out, I was hungry. They were also directly in front of me.

Nyah shot me a perplexed, almost incredulous look. "That stuff's all cheap!" she responded, flipping another drumstick onto the plate. "Lettuce and chicken, that stuff doesn't cost much compared to what I usually buy."

I did a double take. "It was cheaper to eat chicken and salad?" I asked hesitantly. I assumed I'd misunderstood her.

"Yeah." Nyah chuckled. "Actually, I would only spend, like, a hundred and twenty bucks, and then I would have extra food stamps. When I was eating healthy, I would still have extra food stamps throughout the month. Buying bananas, apples, and that stuff is cheap."

"Is it really?" I asked again. I wanted to be sure I was understanding what Nyah was saying. Was she really telling me that healthy food was *less* expensive than unhealthy food?

"Yeah, it's *cheap!*" Nyah reiterated, shooting me a dumbfounded look. Her eyes reflected a growing annoyance at my relentless repetition of the same question. I saw that, but I also couldn't help myself. Nyah was telling me the opposite of everything I'd ever learned about food access and healthy eating.

Now, as I finished entering food budgets into the spreadsheet, our intriguing exchange lingered in my mind. If healthy food was cheap, and Nyah was spending *more* money to get *less* healthy food, then clearly there were other influences beyond price shaping her food choices. And maybe, I thought, those influences affected other families' choices too.

CHAPTER 4

All That Matters

"Miranda?" I asked the towering, stocky woman staring down at her phone. Miranda looked up from her screen and smiled.

"So you're the lady my daughter keeps telling me about," she said, grinning slightly. It was a calm spring evening, and the two of us were meeting outside a busy strip-mall Starbucks.

"Thank you so much for taking the time to meet with me." I reached out, shook Miranda's hand, and asked if I could get her anything to drink. She was in the mood for a strong cup of coffee after a long day at work but politely declined my offer to treat.

"I'll get my drink if you get us a table," she countered, opening the door to the café and letting out a freezing gust of air-conditioning. While Miranda grabbed her coffee, I looked around for a table outside. Options were slim, as high-school students and retirees had parked themselves in patio chairs for the evening, delving into homework or games of checkers. I spotted a small table around the corner that faced the on-ramp to a freeway. The sound of cars accelerating and honking was deafening at first, but as rush hour began to subside, so did the noise.

A few minutes later, Miranda appeared, a small black coffee in hand. She took a seat across from me. At six foot one and just over two hundred pounds, Miranda was a commanding presence. She wore a boxy black short-sleeved T-shirt and billowy jeans. Short, choppy brown hair and a red baseball cap framed a porcelain-white face, and her large hoop earrings swayed back and forth in the breeze. Around her neck hung a gold chain with a heart pendant.

Miranda's intimidating stature was offset by her gentle, soothing voice. It was calming but also so quiet that I feared my audio recorder might not pick up our dialogue over the sound of freeway cars whizzing by. Miranda's seventeen-year-old daughter, Ebony, had spoken in a similar way. I thought back to when I had first met Ebony, two weeks prior. "I'm a vegan," Ebony had disclosed up front. "But I live in a food-insecure home." Ebony's story struck me because it seemed like an outlier or an unusual case. I'd spoken with dozens of kids so far; a low-income kid who also subscribed to a strict diet was, in my experience, rare. So over two cups of green tea at a quiet café one Saturday morning, I'd talked to Ebony to learn how she pulled it off. A few years ago, she told me, she had become a vegan out of a concern for animal welfare. Now she also strongly preferred to eat organic food for environmental and human rights reasons.

While the decision to eat vegan and organic had felt natural, adhering to those preferences had proven challenging. With Miranda's income, Ebony struggled to get the food she needed for a healthy plant-based diet. Ebony's biggest obstacle by far was consuming enough of the foods she really wanted. Not just the ones she needed to survive—like rice and beans—but the foods she craved and that made her feel good and satiated, foods like tofu and almond butter.

"Dates," she answered excitedly when I asked what her favorite food was. The texture, the sweetness, how filling they were— these were the dried fruit's selling points. But, Ebony explained, she rarely ate them.

"They're really expensive," she lamented, tucking a strand of her curly black hair behind her right ear. Tall like her mother, Ebony had a short bob that bounced as she spoke. With a long-sleeved flannel shirt rolled up to her elbows and skinny jeans, she looked comfortable and put together. "I just can't swing it." Ebony let out a sigh of defeat. "My mom can't swing it."

At home with her twin sister, older sister, and mom, Ebony dreamed about a day when she'd be able to afford to stock the fridge with whatever her heart desired. But for the time being, she lived for Fridays. Friday was payday at the health-food store she worked at evenings and weekends, and every Friday, Ebony took her paycheck and treated herself to a trip to her favorite grocery store: Whole Foods.

"It's kind of expensive there," Ebony said, her hands folded neatly on the table. "But it's actually like my favorite store ever."

As much as Ebony relished the smell of fresh tomatoes and basil in the produce section, the vegan sushi rolls filled with cucumber and avocado, and the free kombucha samples, she rarely had the funds to make a trip to Whole Foods worthwhile. The part-time-job paychecks only went so far, and sometimes she had to put her earnings toward household expenses to supplement her mom's earnings. Discount grocers like FoodMaxx and Fresh and Easy were better go-tos for her family's everyday needs.

"I definitely get angry sometimes when there's no food in the house," Ebony said, bringing the steaming mug of tea to her lips. "When you're hungry, you have more of a temper maybe, so when I have to go to school without food, it's annoying."

Even though Ebony qualified for free school meals, the cafeteria had neither vegan nor organic options. Egg and bacon sandwiches, beef tacos, and chicken fingers were on steady rotation, and pickings were slim for non-meat-eaters. Because of this, Ebony largely stayed away from the one place she could easily get free food. Free and reduced-price school meals are meant to provide low-income kids like Ebony with two meals a day five days a week and offset food costs for low-income families. Sometimes, these meals did what they were designed to do; while wealthier kids at Ebony's school congregated in courtyards around colorful lunch boxes and glass containers of food packed at home, most of the low-income kids sat at the long plastic tables inside the cafeteria, light gray trays of school food in front of them. But not every low-income kid. And not Ebony. Most students I spoke with found school meal options repetitive, lackluster, or gross. Many who qualified for the free meals actively tried to avoid them, in part to escape being labeled as poor—the designation that inevitably followed from lining up outside the cafeteria. Together, the low quality and stigma of school meals made them unappealing to the kids they were meant to serve. But when students like Ebony turned these meals down, it put the financial onus back on parents like Miranda to pay for her daughter's meals during the school day.

When the fridge at home was stocked, Ebony brought her own lunches to school. She'd wrap a sandwich in tinfoil or fill a thermos with chili. But sometimes the fridge was empty. In these instances, rather than cave and accept the cafeteria's offerings—and betray her vegan diet—Ebony generally did not eat. She could go six or seven hours with just water, especially if it was carbonated. The little bubbles would fill her stomach, creating the illusion of fullness. Sometimes, when Ebony's hunger pangs grew too intense, she'd grab a piece of unripe fruit from the cafeteria. But more often, she waited until she got home from school and then filled herself up on quinoa. It wasn't her favorite, but it was a healthy, satiating option that she could prepare relatively quickly. Most important, Miranda could afford to buy it in bulk. Every once in a while, the assistant principal at Ebony's school—who knew Ebony came to school hungry most mornings—gave her a gift card to Trader Joe's.

I was eager to hear Miranda's thoughts on Ebony's diet. Originally, Miranda told me, she hadn't been so keen on Ebony's new dietary preferences. But over time, she realized how important veganism was to her daughter, and it became important to her too.

My mind wandered to the stereotypes portraying low-income

moms as unconcerned about their kids' diets. Sitting across from Miranda, I had no doubt that her kids' health and happiness were of the utmost importance to her. She would give—in fact, she had given—anything to support Ebony's choices. Her eyes lit up as she discussed Ebony's love of sauerkraut and soy and all her daughter had taught the family about sustainable seafood. Ebony, Miranda said, beaming, was her "forever teacher."

But something else was equally obvious: Supporting Ebony's choices while also covering the family's living expenses was a relentless struggle and a deep source of stress for Miranda. "Every dime I get goes to pretty much food and bills," Miranda said, leaning back in her chair. "I'm just scraping by."

Until Ebony reached middle school, Miranda had raised her three kids in Bozeman, Montana. It was a nice place, but there were limited opportunities there for a single mom with a GED and line-cook experience. So Miranda moved her kids and then partner, Jenny, out to California so that she could finally realize her longstanding dream of producing and selling cannabis edibles. California was also a place where Miranda, as a white mother, felt more comfortable raising her half-Black children.

Miranda's dream came true when she started working for a small cannabis shop. But unfortunately, the move also prompted Miranda and Jenny to split.

"When Jenny left," Miranda said, "everything kind of went in half." All of a sudden, Miranda was pulling in a fraction of their prior household income. Overnight, she found herself having to say no to virtually everything the kids asked for.

"How come it's always no, no, no?" Ebony and her siblings would complain to their mother. "Money," Miranda told them. "I can't get you anything unless it's free-ninety-nine."

Being poor was hard work. Miranda was one of millions of full-time workers earning a poverty-level wage, or an hourly wage that leaves a full-time, full-year worker below the federal poverty line. Without Jenny, Miranda—despite working fifty or sixty hours per week at the cannabis shop—couldn't carry her family over that line. That made her a member of the working poor, a designation that applies to one in nine full-time employed Americans. Despite breaking their backs, the working poor come up short. Even with a full-time job, Miranda still relied on SNAP to put food on the table and on housing vouchers to pay her rent.

Miranda saw Ebony's new tastes as an additional backbreaking expense. She also felt trapped between her desire to support her daughter and her need to keep the family financially afloat. "When it's someone you love"—she paused, rubbing her necklace between her thumb and index finger—"what do you do?"

What Miranda did was try to make it happen with the paycheck she earned. She was resourceful, shopping around and purchasing older or uglier organic produce untouched by other shoppers. She borrowed a friend's Costco membership to buy in bulk. She started a backyard garden, growing tomatoes and squash. She skipped meals so her kids would have more to eat.

"Sometimes I don't even eat dinner," Miranda told me. "I'll have a bowl of cereal if there is some." She preferred to make sure her kids ate first. "I buy that food for them unless I'm really, *really* hungry.

"The way I feel about food"—Miranda took a final sip of coffee and set the empty paper cup on the table—"is like, if they need food and they're hungry, then I'm gonna buy it. I don't care how much money is in my pocket. I'll spend my last twenty dollars. That's how it is. It'll come. Sometimes it's hard. Everything, literally every dime I get, goes to food. Every dime. But what do you do? I just buy it for them. It's for my babies. I love them more than anything on the planet."

Of course, as with most low-income families, rare moments emerged when Miranda came into a bit of extra money. Maybe she worked some overtime hours or reached into an old coat pocket and found a crumpled bill. Sometimes, it was just a couple of bucks.

"If she wants a two-dollar candy bar," Miranda said about Ebony, "I get it for her if I have it."

But sometimes it was more money, like twenty dollars. When this happened, Miranda said with a grin, she usually gave the cash directly to Ebony to take to the supermarket—even though it felt to Miranda like throwing it away. The other week, she'd given Ebony exactly twenty dollars. With it, Ebony had purchased just two pomelos from Whole Foods.

"Two *pomelos?*" Miranda rolled her eyes. Even now, she couldn't hide her incredulity. It was, she said with a chuckle, just like the story of Jack and the Beanstalk.

In exceptionally rare cases, Miranda found herself with an extra thirty dollars or more. In those moments, her favorite activity involved taking her daughters out to eat. Just a short ride from home was a fancy vegetarian pan-Asian restaurant that Ebony adored. Penny-pinching and saving, Miranda was occasionally able to treat her to a meal there. "Their raw pies are delicious," Miranda noted, a wistful look in her eye. "And we never have leftovers."

Ebony may have been unusual in her dietary preferences, but Miranda reminded me of so many other low-income mothers I had met—the ones who told me that they often spent the last of their paychecks on special meals or foods for their kids. Sometimes, like Miranda, they went out to a big meal with their families or bought pricier items their kids requested. Their accounts didn't fit into the common narrative about low-income families, food access, and nutrition.[1] Their experiences suggested that there was more to the story than public health researchers knew.

Jada Morris, for instance, treated her family of six to luxurious seafood dinners whenever there was enough money in her pocket and enough time to gather the entire family around the table. Once or twice a year, Jada would take a hearty chunk of her SNAP benefits for the month and splurge on fresh crab, lobster, and scallops. The weekend before I sat down with her, she had spent eighty-five dollars on six crabs.

"I was like, we're gonna eat good today." Jada laughed. "I took those crabs and cleaned them and boiled them and I fried them. And the kids, they ate them all up, and it was good."

The purchase had put Jada in the hole for the next month, but she didn't mind. "It was worth it," she said, a satisfied grin sweeping across her face. "The rest of my stamps I have to save for Thanksgiving. I can't spend no more. Have to make do with what we have now."

After wrapping up my interview with Miranda, I sat in my car for half an hour scribbling random thoughts and ideas in my notebook. I kept returning to one central source of confusion. *I thought it was all about money,* I wrote. *But if that's true, then I can't explain some of these food purchases.*

If Miranda was spending a paycheck on a family dinner at a restaurant while also struggling to make rent, then her food choices couldn't be solely financially motivated. Miranda clearly didn't *always* prioritize spending the absolute least amount of money on food. Sometimes she did, but other times she didn't. The same was true for Jada—and Nyah too. As influential as food prices were to moms, I realized something else wielded incredible influence: Their kids' desires. Their kids' happiness.

Miranda strove to buy food with the best financial value, but she was also trying to secure food with the most *symbolic* value to her kids.[2]

Spending thirty dollars or more on one restaurant dinner was a lot for Miranda. She rarely had that kind of money lying around, and she could certainly have found other uses for it— that was enough money to restock the family's quinoa and bean supply or pay for a week's utilities. But what didn't make sense financially for Miranda made perfect sense symbolically. A meal out gave Miranda the opportunity to bring a genuine smile to

Ebony's face—to surprise and delight her. A meal out gave Miranda a moment out of her busy schedule to sit and connect with her daughter over delicious, warm, and satiating food. A meal out offered Miranda a chance to show Ebony that she was listening—that she really heard and would do anything to honor her daughter's preferences. A meal out gave Miranda the rare chance to say yes to Ebony.

Those nights when Miranda could treat Ebony to a special meal reminded her that amid all the hardship—amid the empty kitchen cupboards and the growl of her own stomach most evenings as she climbed into bed—she was still a loving and capable mother. For all that, thirty dollars was a steal.

"They want food, they'll get it," Miranda told me about her children. "One day they'll know. They'll know I love them, and that's all that matters."

PART II

Nourishment

Even after all this time
The sun never says to the earth
"You owe me."
Look what happens with a love like that
It lights the whole sky
— DANIEL LADINSKY, "EVEN AFTER ALL THIS TIME"

CHAPTER 5

Scarcity, Abundance

On a blistering-hot Monday afternoon in June, I sat on the worn beige couch in Nyah Baker's garage. The garage door was open to the driveway and sunlight poured into the concrete room. Next to me, Nyah leaned forward on a light gray polyester recliner with Natasha cross-legged at her feet. For the past hour, Nyah had been braiding Natasha's hair, weaving in thick black wig strands to create a voluminous braid. The two of them passed a green Costco-size bag of pistachios back and forth every few minutes, each taking small handfuls.

Earlier that morning, I'd texted Nyah to figure out what time I should come by. When I didn't hear back for a few hours, I figured she was otherwise occupied. Nyah was often busy with her daughters rather than glued to her phone. So I hopped in my car and drove down to her place. When I stepped out onto her street a half hour later, the still, hot air enveloped me.

Nyah's neighbors were mostly Mexican-American and Black families, the majority of whom were low-income. Black families were a shrinking minority in the Bay Area. From 1970 to 2010, the region's Black population declined from 13.8 percent to 7 percent. Gentrification, rising rental costs, and federal and local exclusionary policies displaced Black communities while also keeping them out of whiter neighborhoods. As a result, many Black families were driven to the Bay Area's outer reaches.[1]

But in this particular neighborhood, Nyah, Nyah's sister, and dozens of other Black families had managed to stay put.

I waved hello to Marcus, Nyah's boyfriend, who was fixing up his van at the edge of her driveway, squatting to fill a back tire with air. I heard Simon, their football-size mutt, yapping away in the backyard that wrapped around Nyah's house like a moat. As usual, the garage door was open, and I spotted Nyah and Natasha settling in for an afternoon of hairstyling. Nyah used to have air-conditioning in the house, but last summer, after Nyah had been repeatedly late paying her bills, the landlord had removed the AC unit. Without that indoor respite from the blazing heat, the garage was now the airiest spot available to the Bakers. The radio blasted nineties jams, and Nyah had engineered a breeze by tilting a standing fan in their direction.

"Did you text me sometime in the past couple days?" Nyah asked as I strolled up the driveway, using my hand as a visor to block the sun. In her solid pink tank top and checkered pink boxer shorts, she was dressed for the weather. I mentioned my text earlier that morning, and she nodded. Her and the girls' phones had all been turned off the past few days because she hadn't had the money to pay that month's phone bill. The bills were due on the twenty-fifth of each month. Today was the twenty-seventh.

"But I just got some money yesterday," Nyah assured me, pulling a coarse black strand of Natasha's hair taut. "We can all go pay it off today."

I sat on the couch as Nyah and I caught up from the weekend. Nyah had visited a friend who lived about forty minutes north. The friend had loaned Nyah enough gas money for her to make the journey. They ate subs and drank beer. Overall, Nyah said, it wasn't a bad time.

"What are you up to for the Fourth of July?" I asked her, sliding deeper into the couch, aware that this might be my seat for the next couple of hours. Nyah was planning to take the kids to

Fresno—a three-hour drive—to camp with the rest of her family. Nyah's brothers and sisters all lived within a few hours of one another, and it was a tradition for them to get together with the kids on Independence Day. But with her car's air-conditioning busted for the past three months, Nyah was dreading the car trip.

"It's hard because I'm heavy," Nyah explained. "And that makes it really hot to sit in that car." Having spent a good amount of time personally stuck to its sunbaked leather seats, I could see what Nyah meant. While Nyah waited on Marcus to find and install a new unit, the last thing any of us wanted to do on a day like today was pile inside those four doors.

Still, Nyah was keen on heading to Fresno because it would likely be her last big trip before her hysterectomy. She wanted to make it count.

"I just really want to go camping before I have to have my surgery," she said, letting out a tired sigh and handing Natasha the bag of pistachios. For the past few months, Nyah had been suffering. Her uterus had grown increasingly inflamed, and the growing fibroids made her writhe in pain. That pain was overshadowed only by Nyah's fears about undergoing major surgery with general anesthesia. Nyah wasn't sure she'd survive being put under, which was one reason why this Fourth of July trip felt so important. Maybe it would be her last time with her family. And Nyah needed the boost; not being able to work this summer had taken its toll on her mental health.

"I want to work," she said, frowning. "It's just the health stuff that's like a block. It's like a wall stopping me."

Nyah took medication to cope with the stress that came with not having a steady income. She also had pills to calm anxiety attacks, two of which she'd experienced in the past month alone. The weekly visits to her psychiatrist helped, but Nyah knew her challenges fell outside the scope of his expertise. One day she'd feel fine, the next she'd spiral down. The drugs helped bring her back, but they rarely stopped her from eventually swinging to the other end of the pendulum.

"You never know what you're gonna get with me." Nyah rolled her eyes, leaned back in the lounger, and cracked her knuckles to ease the tension from braiding Natasha's hair.

This summer, Nyah felt more frustrated and bored than she had in years. She felt frustrated because money was scarcer than ever and bored because that scarcity limited her and the girls' possibilities. When she'd been working, Nyah had been able to cover the rent and utilities and still have enough left over to take Mariah and Natasha to the water park. Now, with no steady income and barely enough to cover the essentials, Nyah didn't have the funds she needed to make the most of summer for her girls.

"The thing is," Nyah told me, "you need money to do stuff."

"Priya's here!" I heard Jane yell to her mom. It was a sunny Tuesday afternoon in September, and I was standing outside the Cains' front door. I could hear the doorbell sounding through the house and their collie Max's paws slipping and sliding on the living-room floor. Julie's footsteps trailed behind him.

"Come on in!" Julie said after she opened the door and greeted me with a bright smile. Dressed in skinny jeans and a gray T-shirt, she looked ready to go out, save for the fuzzy slippers she wore to keep her feet warm on the hardwood floors.

I slipped off my flats in the entryway; Max rolled over at my feet and I knelt down to scratch his stomach. I'd obliged him the first time we met, and he'd remembered ever since. I made my way into the kitchen and found Jane in black leggings and a black T-shirt, ready for dance class. She was sitting on a stool at the granite island with a jar of Planter's peanuts in one hand. Every couple of minutes, she reached the other hand into the container and pulled out a few nuts.

There was an abundance of food on display in the Cains'

kitchen. A large fruit bowl overflowed with navel oranges, clementines, mandarins, and limes, and a two-tiered basket was filled with bananas, butternut squash, peaches, and onions. To the right of the sink, neatly laid out, were all the Trader Joe's ingredients for that evening's dinner: a bag of tortilla chips, avocado, black beans, refried beans, chili-lime spice, and gluten-free tortillas.

"Taco Tuesday!" Julie smiled as she saw me eyeing the ingredients.

While Julie organized some papers on the dining-room table, I plopped myself down on the stool beside Jane, and we chatted about her two favorite after-school activities: dance and volleyball.

Earlier that day, Julie had texted me our agenda for the afternoon. The plan was to spend that afternoon, like many afternoons, shuttling the kids around. In a few minutes, we'd drop Jane off at the dance studio. While she was there, Julie and I would go to the bank, pick up dry cleaning, and then stop by home for a little bit to relax. Afterward, we'd get Jane and bring her home again so that she could change and grab a snack, then we'd drive Jane to volleyball camp, come back home, and make dinner for everyone. Julie and I would eat with Evan; Zach would collect Jane on his way home from work, and the two of them would have a late dinner. Maybe, Julie joked, they'd even clean up.

Sometimes when I was with Julie, amid all of the picking up and dropping off, my mind would wander. I'd think of my afternoons with Nyah. I'd recall the feeling of watching TV while sinking deeper and deeper into the couch. As parents, Nyah and Julie had very different lives.

"Mom, it's time to go." Jane jumped up, screwed the lid back onto the peanut jar, and put it away in the cupboard. Julie nodded, grabbing her purse from the counter. As Julie refilled her reusable water bottle, she asked Jane if she had remembered her own water bottle.

"Yup," Jane said, heading toward the garage. "But I'm not going to take a granola bar because I'm not going to be doing that much." Julie nodded approvingly, pulling out her keys from her purse.

Today, the conversation in the car was a bit stilted. Jane sat in the back seat of the Cains' Mercedes, her eyes glued to her phone. From the driver's seat, Julie threw questions toward the back—"How was school today?" "How is social studies class going?"—that Jane grudgingly answered with one-syllable responses.

At first, I wondered if I was the reason for the silence. Perhaps I made everyone feel self-conscious or uncomfortable. But Julie had assured me earlier that that's what Jane did now. Her world was in her phone.

That afternoon, though, Jane wasn't just quiet. This was something more, I realized. She was in a bad mood.

"Do you need a tutor for math?" Julie gently asked her daughter, flipping the left blinker on as we pulled into the dance studio's parking lot.

"I'm fine, Mom," Jane said as she continued tapping on her screen. Her irritation was palpable. Jane explained that she had gotten a twenty-five out of thirty on a math quiz a week ago, but she had improved her score to a twenty-six out of thirty on the next quiz. Julie hoped to continue the conversation, but Jane made it clear that they were done for now, swinging open the car door and hopping out onto the concrete.

An hour later, when we picked Jane up from dance, her mood seemed to have worsened. After a quick pit stop at home, we made the forty-five-minute drive to volleyball camp. The three of us sat in silence the entire ride.

"Have a good time!" Julie yelled cheerfully to Jane as she slid the back door open and climbed out. Jane responded with only a forced grin before slamming the door shut and disappearing into the gym.

As we looped around the parking lot, I was struck by Julie's silence. Usually, she was chatty when it was just the two of us in the car. She'd tell me stories from the weekend or update me on her kids. But now, Julie seemed upset, and she didn't have to tell me why. I knew it had to do with Jane. For ten minutes, I joined Julie in silence. We each sat absorbed in our own thoughts, the muffled voices of an NPR newscast playing faintly in the background.

"You know," Julie eventually said, glancing in my direction as we pulled up to a stoplight, "Jane has basically always gotten everything she wants."

Judging from the time I'd spent with the Cains, I thought that assertion rang true. I was starting to get Jane's world; it was one where so much of what she asked for was not only possible, but usually granted. Whether Jane wanted front-row seats to a Beyoncé concert, new Lululemon leggings, or plane tickets to fly across the country and visit family, Julie and Zach almost always seemed able and willing to say yes. But Jane didn't always seem to appreciate just how good she had it. When Julie and Zach had given Jane those Beyoncé tickets for her birthday, Jane asked them what else they'd gotten her.

"She lives in a bubble," Julie explained. "And if I'm honest, she's really spoiled."

Again, my mind drifted to Mariah and Natasha. Any of the gifts Jane had received were beyond their wildest dreams. Beyond their mom's too. It seemed to me, in that moment, at that stoplight, that Julie's and Nyah's worlds had never been farther apart.

As moms, Julie and Nyah shared simple truths: they loved their children more than anything, and they found raising them to be both immensely joyful and, at times, terribly stressful. Both knew intimately that nurturing kids was filled with struggles and triumphs and that it was at once an immediate challenge and a long-term investment. As their kids had slowly grown into teenagers, both moms had watched their maturation in awe while also missing the days when their babies would snuggle into their laps and stare up admiringly into their eyes.

While these shared emotions bound Julie and Nyah, their tangible experiences as moms diverged sharply.

To my eye, these diverging experiences seemed to be largely the consequence of the different contexts within which Nyah and Julie were raising their kids. And yet I struggled to pinpoint exactly what accounted for their vastly different parenting experiences. What specifically widened the gulf between them? Was it the different neighborhoods the Cains and the Bakers lived in, the different homes they shared with their families, the different schools their kids attended, or their different household incomes? Was it the fact that Julie navigated the world as a married, white, affluent woman and Nyah as a single, Black, low-income one? When it came to their parenting experiences, how much did it matter that Julie's family had few, if any, financial stresses while Nyah was living so close to the bone? Which of these differences mattered a great deal, which ones mattered somewhat, and which ones didn't matter at all?

My job as a sociologist was to zero in on each of these factors—Julie's and Nyah's distinct neighborhoods, incomes, and racial identities—and explain how each specifically affected their families' diets. But trying to isolate these kinds of individual factors and quantify their precise impacts proved fruitless. No *one* factor could adequately account for how widely—profoundly, even—Julie's and Nyah's paths diverged.

Yes, Julie's and Nyah's neighborhoods differed. Yes, they had different housing situations. Yes, their financial circumstances were light-years apart, and yes, they had vastly different degrees of racial and socioeconomic privilege. But as I interrogated each of these differences, I came to appreciate that each difference individually mattered in large part because of what it contributed to the whole. Together, *all* of these differences coalesced into distinct holistic parenting experiences. They created, essentially, different worlds for Julie and Nyah.

Julie had many resources that eased the grind of motherhood. She had money, time, security, stability, and the safety of white privilege. The accumulation of these assets meant that Julie parented in relative comfort. The Cain kids may have had their issues (what teenagers didn't?) but there was never any question as to whether their basic needs would be met. Julie did not worry about whether Jane and Evan had the essential necessities to carry on physically and emotionally. Nyah, on the other hand, couldn't always take that for granted. In fact, she rarely could. While Nyah had time, that was about all she shared with Julie. She worried about keeping the lights on, the fridge stocked, and her kids out of the police's gaze. Nyah often felt one step away from her daughters not having enough—of them not being okay.

Nyah parented in a world of scarcity. Julie did so in a world of abundance. And this deeper fault line dividing Julie and Nyah as parents, I discovered, shaped food's dramatically different meanings to each of them.

CHAPTER 6

Within Reach

One afternoon, Nyah thought she might come into some money. We'd gone out to pay off the cell phone bills and grab six dollars' worth of glazed and powdered doughnuts, and we were in the Dunkin' Donuts parking lot when a call came in. Nyah had looked down at the unknown number, furrowing her brow before answering with a quiet, suspicious "Yes?" The man on the other end congratulated her on being eligible to receive seven thousand dollars from the federal government, no strings attached. Nyah asked to borrow my pen and notebook to write some information down. I handed them over, and she quickly scribbled a few words and numbers on a blank page. After hanging up the phone a few minutes later, Nyah ripped the sheet of paper out of my notebook, folded it up, and stuffed it in her purse. Turning to me, she explained that the man had said she could pick up the money at Walmart anytime.

"I thought it was a scam at first," Nyah said, popping a powdered doughnut hole into her mouth. But then she considered that maybe it was legitimate.

"I'm sure going to try it." Nyah rolled her eyes, a slight grin crossing her face. "Broke like I am."

Ultimately, though, Nyah didn't try it. Back at the house later that afternoon, Nyah called a friend who warned her that it wasn't a good idea. "She's right," Nyah told me. "Plus, they told me that first I needed to buy a card for two hundred and thirty dollars before I could get the seven thousand." She paused. "I think it's a scam."

During the months I spent at Nyah's side, that was neither the first nor the last time she would be called with an enticing but ultimately spurious offer. Nyah was a consistent target of phone scams. Some were initially exciting, like when she learned about different prizes she'd won, low-interest loans she'd qualified for, or new government benefits she'd earned. Others were scarier, like when she was informed that her Social Security number had been hacked or she was going to be arrested for fraud. Most calls ended with a request for her credit card number, at which point Nyah would crack up. "You think I use a credit card?" She'd chuckle and hang up.

Still, Nyah approached each call with cautious optimism. As unlikely as it was, maybe one of them would turn out to be the real deal. "You only gotta win the lottery once," she'd say, a soft chuckle escaping her lips.

But Nyah never won the lottery. Her time never came. Days, weeks, and months went by. We passed them in her garage, where we sat immersed in sitcoms and movies from the early 2000s. As Nyah spoke to the friend who told her that the seven-thousand-dollar offer was probably a scam, we were watching our second movie of the day, the 2004 remake of *Walking Tall*, which starred Natasha's all-time-favorite actor and celebrity crush, the Rock. Then Mariah came by and the sisters played on their phones while Nyah and Marcus cracked open two cans of Bud Light that Marcus had bought at the gas station three blocks away. Their next-door neighbors Jim and Big Mike—two white, burly mechanics with tattoos and a few hours to kill— stopped by to say hi and bum a couple of cigarettes off Marcus.

The afternoon dragged on. Our foreheads glistened in the summer heat. My eyes began to glaze over as one movie bled into another. We passed around a roll of Ritz crackers while Nyah worked carefully and meticulously on Natasha's hair.

It's almost like Nyah is drawing out the time, I scribbled in my notebook. *It's like she's trying to fill the hours and minutes to get to the end of the day.*

The highlight of that afternoon came as the clock hit six and I could hear, at first faintly, the recognizable jingle of an ice cream truck. The truck was making its way through the neighborhood, and its music intensified as it rounded the block onto Nyah's street. Finally, out of the corner of my eye, I spotted it three houses down.

"Stop the truck!" Nyah bellowed at Marcus, who had planted himself on the side of the road to repair a friend's motorcycle. "Stop it so Natty can get an ice cream!" Nyah yelled again. Natty, as Natasha was affectionately called, hadn't asked her mom for an ice cream. In fact, she'd been so engrossed in the movie that she'd hardly noticed the truck nearby. But as Marcus flagged it down, Nyah tapped on Natasha's shoulder, and she stood up, her hand outstretched toward her mom. Nyah dug into her purse and pulled out two crinkled dollar bills. She smoothed them out with her fingers and laid the bills in Natasha's hand. Then she looked at me. "You want anything?" she asked, as she often did whenever she bought her daughters anything. Nyah never let poverty diminish her hospitality or her humanity.

"No, I'm okay." I smiled. "But I'll go with Natasha to see what they're selling." Natasha and I hustled down to the end of the driveway just as the ice cream truck slowed to a halt. Natasha quickly scanned the menu on the side of the truck before ordering Airheads Xtremes Sweetly Sour Candy Belts. From the image on the carton, the candies looked like miniature rainbow conveyor belts coated in frosty sugar.

That's really smart, I thought. *Better to get something that won't instantly melt in this blazing heat.*

We walked back up to the house and Natasha resumed her position at Nyah's feet so her mom could continue with the hair weave. Natasha opened the carton, pulled out a strip, and handed it behind her head to Nyah. Nyah took a bite and paused.

"Mmm." She nodded, savoring the bite. "That's good!"

The three of us sat there for a couple more hours as the sun dipped behind neighbors' houses and the air cooled. Nyah nursed a beer, and I followed the plot of another Rock movie. Mariah left to meet up with friends and came back with a carton of McDonald's fries and a medium Coke for her little sister. Sharing the fries, the two of them perched side by side on the couch as the opening credits for another thriller scrolled across the screen.

It was a day like any other day that summer. If I were to ask Nyah about any of it now, I doubt she'd remember it.

Little happened. That was the point. The deeper I sank into Nyah's couch, the more keenly I noticed something. As stressful as financial scarcity was, it could also be tedious. It could make daily life monotonous. With nowhere to go and nothing to do, Nyah had little she could give to Mariah and Natasha that they would get excited about.

What's more, with no signs of income on the way, there wasn't a lot to look forward to. The next morning, the sun would again rise, and the girls would resume their positions on the couch. This time, Nyah would style Mariah's hair. Someone else would call with an offer of seven thousand dollars or more, the neighbors would come over, and the ice cream truck would once again roll around the corner. The days would pass, but Nyah never seemed to have the financial means to take advantage of them. She had time, sure. But without money, she and her daughters were stuck in that garage.

One evening in early June, Nyah had sat Mariah and Natasha down to mentally prepare them for the long summer ahead. Trying to spin a difficult situation into a positive lesson, she explained to her daughters that despite all that they lacked, there was still a great deal to be thankful for. Nyah knew that it was a hard sell, and she felt bad about it. But what if she could help *them* not feel so bad about it?

"I told them it's not all about fancy clothes and fancy cars," Nyah recounted to me. "'Be happy you have a roof over your head, you have food in here, you can watch TV when you want to and use the bathroom whenever you want to. You have a fan inside to go to when you get hot, and a blanket to get under when you're cold.'" After Nyah relayed this story to me, she paused for a moment, glancing down at the phone in her right hand.

"I'm just trying to survive," she whispered, looking back up to meet my eyes.

Surviving came with sacrifices. And like other parents, Nyah survived and saved money by consistently saying no to her children's large requests.

I thought about Julie, who had the means to parent in a constant flow of yes—yes to the big things like private school and dance classes and yes to the smaller things like a new pair of shoes and a replacement for a shattered phone screen. In contrast, Nyah had to say no to her kids constantly. Summer camp was off the table, as was a trip to Disneyland or even a day pass to the local water park. Even the smaller things—a trendy pair of jeans or a refurbished iPad—were off the table. None of these were indulgences that Nyah could provide on her budget.

Nyah's constantly having to say no wasn't just hard on Mariah and Natasha; it was also devastating and guilt-inducing for Nyah herself. It made her feel less-than.

And yet, next to all the things Nyah truly couldn't afford, food was different. More often than not, food was miraculously within reach. Unlike larger items like new sweaters or even grander indulgences like family vacations, gifts of food were actually within the realm of possibility for Nyah. Almost always, Nyah had a few dollars lying around. She could generally overturn a sofa cushion or plunge her hand into her purse and scrounge up a buck and a handful of coins. That money was never enough to pay off a bill or fill up a gas tank, but that didn't mean it was useless.

It had value because it could help Nyah say yes to her daughters' junk-food requests. On a daily basis, food was *the* thing she and her girls could afford and the thing they could look forward to. A one-dollar doughnut, a two-dollar ice cream, a three-dollar burger, Airheads Xtremes Sweetly Sour Candy Belts. These were treats Nyah could swing that brought smiles to her daughters' faces. So on a recent trip to the grocery store when Natasha asked Nyah for a ninety-nine-cent bag of Doritos, Nyah said yes. When Mariah requested a dollar-fifty Dr Pepper, Nyah obliged. These small purchases were what allowed Nyah to say yes to her kids at least once a day.

Just because Nyah said yes to her girls' junk-food requests didn't mean that she didn't care about their health. Nyah talked often about how good nutrition was key to her and her daughters' health. One afternoon, as Nyah, Mariah, and I drove to the pawnshop, Nyah monologued about the importance of a nutritious diet for longevity. Mariah sat in the front seat eating Fruity Pebbles out of the box, singing along to the radio while gobbling up handfuls of the colorful, puffy balls. Glancing at her daughter, Nyah said matter-of-factly, "If you eat well, you're going to live long, that's for sure."

Another afternoon, Nyah told me that she didn't really want the girls to be eating junk food. "Some things they do ask me, and I don't like to buy that stuff for them." Nyah let out a heavy sigh, then added, "They win. They win all the time."

Food for her girls is where I most often saw Nyah's money go. One Saturday, we'd ducked into a hole-in-the-wall salon where Nyah paid twenty-eight dollars to get her and her daughters' eyebrows threaded. Of the many hours I'd spent at her side, that was one of the few non-food-related activities I saw Nyah take her kids to. Most of the time, she was spending a few dollars here and a few dollars there on small edible treats.

What if Nyah just saved her money? This was a question I asked myself often, not because I thought she should, but because I knew someone would eventually fire it at me. This seemed like an almost inevitable outcome of sharing my observations more widely. Critics would point out how financially irrational parents like Nyah acted, how frivolously she wasted what little money she had. If Nyah had just saved all of the cash that she spent on cans of Sprite and Wendy's chicken sandwiches, they'd argue, maybe she could lift herself out of poverty. If Nyah was in dire straits but also squandering her money on junk food rather than investing or saving it, then she had no one to blame but herself.

The idea that low-income people like Nyah are responsible for their position below the poverty line is known as the culture-of-poverty argument. The theory originated in the 1960s with the anthropologist Oscar Lewis. Lewis argued that sustained poverty generated a set of cultural attitudes, beliefs, values, and practices, and that this culture of poverty would likely perpetuate itself over time, even if the structural conditions that gave rise to it changed. Lewis's idea was popularized by the sociologist Daniel Patrick Moynihan, then an assistant labor secretary to Lyndon B. Johnson, who introduced the idea to the public in 1965 in what became known as the Moynihan Report. Moynihan argued that Black families were caught in a "tangle of pathology" that resulted from the cumulative effects of slavery and structural poverty. In particular, he blamed Black poverty on "ghetto culture," failure to marry, and absent Black fathers.

Moynihan's argument quickly gained steam among conservatives. It furthered the idea that people in poverty played a central role in maintaining and reproducing their conditions, and it also reinforced racist stereotypes about Black communities' loose family morals. It was up to Black people, conservatives opined, to extricate *themselves* from a perpetuating cycle of poverty.

The culture-of-poverty argument has been the subject of much backlash, with critics underscoring how it diverts attention away from structural barriers and toward blaming the victim. Social scientists have shown that poor individuals don't have different or "delinquent" values that perpetuate their circumstances; rather, they face systemic obstacles that cement them and their children in place. Sociologists like Mario Small and Michèle Lamont have worked to refine what *culture* is and isn't and how it interacts with structures to reproduce inequality and limit social mobility. But the argument still circulates, reinforcing an American individualistic viewpoint that people should be able to pull themselves up by their bootstraps. As recently as 2020, Lawrence Mead, a professor of politics and public policy, published an article titled "Poverty and Culture" in which he argued that neither racism nor policy failures were responsible for poverty in the United States. Rather, the long-term poor themselves—namely, Black and Latinx people—lacked the individualism, ambition, and "enterprising temperament" of descendants of European immigrants.[1] (Following scholarly outcry and condemnations of the piece as "false, prejudicial, and stigmatizing," the journal that published the article, *Society*, retracted it.[2])

In light of this intellectual history, I knew that my research observations could be interpreted in wildly different ways. I shuddered at the thought that, taken out of context, what I had observed could mistakenly be seen as buttressing a culture-of-poverty argument. By truthfully showing where Nyah chose to put her money, might I inadvertently bolster a view that she was responsible for the hardships she endured? Might my findings suggest that Nyah's spending choices were what kept her in poverty? Worst of all, might they reinforce racist tropes of single, Black moms as lazy or irresponsible?

This was completely counter to my aims. And yet I couldn't lie about what I had observed; as a scientist, I had an ethical obligation to present my observations as fully and transparently as they'd transpired before my eyes.

But, I realized, I also had the profound responsibility to put these observations into the correct context.

So yes, it was true that I'd seen Nyah spend six dollars on doughnuts, seven on chicken fingers and fries, and ten on Frappuccinos. But there was also this truth: even if Nyah didn't spend that money on her kids, twenty-three dollars wouldn't lift her out of poverty. It wouldn't change her circumstances. With the number of debt collectors coming by, the bills to pay, unexpected medical expenses, and family emergencies, that money was going out the door no matter what. It always did. I'd seen Nyah's last bills fly out of her wallet—fifty bucks to help a friend pay for a funeral, forty to help make another's bail, twenty to pay off her sister's cell phone bill, forty-five to keep her own daughters' phones working. There was always a debt to pay and someone coming around to collect it.

The author and activist James Baldwin once said, "Anyone who has ever struggled with poverty knows how extremely expensive it is to be poor." Nyah's life was testament to this truth. Nyah spent a significant share of what little money she had to keep herself and her kids housed and safe. First, when Nyah was working, she put over half of her income toward her rent, making her "severely rent-burdened" like one in every five Americans. Even with all she paid for housing, there were additional expenses that added to her monthly bills, expenses I didn't see high-income families dealing with. For instance, the water from Nyah's kitchen faucet wasn't safe to drink, so she spent around forty dollars each month on bottled water for her family, although sometimes Nyah would drink the tap water and save the bottles for her daughters. Nyah also paid for a security system—eighteen dollars a month—after her house was broken into twice in three months, an expense that families in safer neighborhoods didn't have.

I also saw how consistently coming up short—how never having any financial reserves to draw from—*increased* Nyah's expenses. Her jewelry was one example. Years ago, when Nyah lost her job, she didn't have enough to make rent. That week, she pawned what jewelry she had for two hundred dollars, which allowed her to keep a roof over her and her daughters' heads. As the months wore on, Nyah wanted to get the jewelry back, but the cost of pulling the jewelry out of the pawnshop also increased. She never had the two hundred forty dollars she needed to get it out, so she continued to pay a storage fee of sorts—thirty-five dollars a month, which came to more than four hundred dollars a year—for the shop to keep holding on to it.

There are other examples of how expensive poverty is. Nyah couldn't afford a newer car, which meant that she was constantly forking over money to repair her old one. She didn't have enough money at any moment to put in the bank to gain interest, making her one of the nine million Americans without a bank account. She was constantly paying late fees. Five years earlier, Nyah had gotten a credit card but failed to pay the monthly bill when she needed to redirect her money toward buying a new car part so she could drive to work. Then the interest started compounding and Nyah could never get on top of it. She still owed the credit card company tens of thousands of dollars.

"They be callin', harassing and threatening me," Nyah explained. "I'm like, 'Whatever. I'm already broke.'" Nyah knew she'd never pay that card off or qualify for a credit card ever again. Having no reserves and no support made climbing out of poverty an impossibility.

That knowledge shaped how Nyah dealt with money when she had it. Dollar bills were ephemeral, best suited for spending before someone took them away again.

I could see how Nyah's decision to spend rather than save

might seem irrational. But rationality is always subject to context. What is irrational in one context may be highly rational in another.

As I saw cash fly in and out of Nyah's hands, I understood that a context of financial scarcity and instability made Nyah's junk-food spending the most rational choice in the world. Nyah spent the money in her pocket on her kids—what the sociologist Allison Pugh calls "windfall child rearing"—because it wasn't clear how empty or full her pocket might be the next day.[3] Nyah used cash on hand like the windfall it was—a piece of good luck, its presence not to be taken for granted or assumed in the future. Money now did not mean money later. For Nyah, the decision to treat the girls came down to the fact that she couldn't know when another emergency might strike or another bill collector would call. If Nyah didn't treat her kids today, she might not have anything to give Mariah and Natasha for weeks. That was not okay. Good moms made sacrifices to give their kids joy. Good moms found a way when there was no way.[4]

Nyah found a way, and that way was saying yes to her daughters whenever it was possible. Nyah generally prioritized satisfying the girls' immediate wants for chips, soda, and candy rather than risk losing the chance to get them anything at all. This was how Nyah made lemonade out of the bitter lemons she'd been given. It was how she provided for her girls, knowing they'd likely never have all the opportunities she wanted for them. Those opportunities were, she felt, off the table. But food wasn't.

CHAPTER 7

Being "Good"

The first time I met Dana Williams, she and I chatted at one of a handful of wooden tables inside a supermarket. We sat kitty-corner from each other, the smell of pastrami and pasta salad from the deli just a few feet away filling our noses. During the conversation, Dana's thirteen-year-old daughter, Madison, kept herself entertained by touring the grocery aisles. Madison stopped by our table five times over the course of an hour with various goodies: gummies, Ritz crackers, tortilla chips, chocolate-covered pretzels, soda.

"Can I have this?" she asked her mom each time, smiling hopefully while holding the treat up with one hand. Dana explained that Madison could pick one. As her daughter walked away, Dana turned to me.

"I feel bad," she said, letting out a heavy sigh. "But I'm a single mom. I can't get her everything she wants."

This was neither the first nor the last time I would watch Madison and her younger sister, Paige, beg their mom for junk food. One Wednesday evening, I met Dana at her house to join her family for a grocery run to Target. I was hanging out on the front stoop with Dana's mom, Debra, and the two girls when Dana got home feeling exhausted, as she did most evenings. In her medical-assistant scrubs, she trudged up the driveway with her purse and a thermos of water, a tired look in her eyes. Madison and Paige, in contrast, were bursting with energy. Paige ran up to Dana and threw her pudgy arms around her mom's waist. Dana put her hand on Paige's back and bent over to kiss the top of her head. Madison stood up on the front steps.

"Can we go to Target now?" she asked her mom, a hand on one hip.

"Don't I get a hello?" Dana said, feigning offense.

"Hello," Madison said in a deadpan tone, the sides of her mouth beginning to curl slightly upward to reveal a grin.

"Hello." Dana matched Madison's tone. We all broke into grins.

"They've been asking to go all day," Debra told her daughter, pulling a pack of cigarettes out of her jeans pocket and taking a few steps away from everyone to light one. "But I told them they had to wait till Mom got home."

Dana nodded. I could tell from the ever-present bags under her eyes and the way she'd dragged her feet coming up the driveway that the last thing Dana wanted to do was head back out. As she often did within five minutes of getting home, Dana wanted to change out of her scrubs into yoga pants and a tank top and then plop herself down on the couch, put her feet up, flip through pictures on her phone, and catch up on the day with Debra. But the only thing Dana hated more than going back out after work was letting Madison and Paige down, so the five of us loaded ourselves into Dana's Honda Civic.

Inside Target, families roamed brightly lit, well-stocked aisles. Dads pushed around carts filled with jumbo packs of toilet paper, and kids pulled at moms' pant legs, begging for video games, baseball caps, and Snickers bars. As we began our stroll through the grocery department, Paige and Madison started begging Dana for what felt like everything in sight. They pointed out virtually every appetizing item they spotted: Velveeta mac and cheese. Extra-large marshmallows. Cinnamon Toast Crunch. Taco shells. If I hadn't known they were *asking* for these items, I would have assumed they were giving us a tour of the supermarket or practicing reading labels.

But they weren't docents of a grocery excursion; they had an agenda. We hadn't been in the cookie and cereal aisle for two minutes before Paige's index finger shot up toward the top shelf.

"Mom, cinnamon-roll Oreos with peanut butter!" she yelled, teetering on her tiptoes to get a better view. Dana ignored Paige as she rolled her shopping cart over to the juice section. Dana's strategy for moving forward without getting stalled, I quickly learned, was to pretend she couldn't hear her daughters. This only sort of worked. Dana ignored the girls, and the girls ignored Dana ignoring them. Paige grabbed a bag of pancake mix to show Dana, and Madison yelled out, "Cinnamon Pop-Tarts!" We chose a chocolate powder for Madison to mix with milk in the morning for breakfast as Paige screamed in the background, "Mom, can we please get cereal? I am begging you!" Dana allowed the girls to put items in the cart. Then she stealthily removed those items once her daughters were distracted with something else.

This back-and-forth continued as we navigated the eight aisles of food and drinks. Halfway through, Dana turned to me and said, exasperation palpable in her voice, "As you can imagine, I prefer to grocery shop by myself." She pulled a box of Cookie Crisp cereal out of the shopping cart and put it back on the shelf. "They have way too much energy."

When it came to food marketing, the supermarket aisles were a battlefield. Everywhere we looked, there were packages meant to appeal to both kids and parents. So many foods that Paige and Madison begged for were designed to make kids' mouths water and simultaneously assuage parents' guilt about buying them. The Cocoa Puffs box was a great example. Madison's and Paige's eyes were drawn to the cute cartoon bird drinking chocolate milk through a straw from a heaping bowl of crunchy brown puffs next to the words *Cuckoo for Chocolatey Milk!* That imagery, combined with the brown background, screamed *chocolate*. But at the top of the box was the comforting message *With Whole Grain First Ingredient,* meant to assure moms that this unhealthy-looking cereal was actually a nutritious choice for their kids—or at least that it wasn't complete junk. The Kraft macaroni-and-cheese box struck this same balance, highlighting for kids how completely cheesy and comforting the package's contents were while at the same time assuring parents that the product contained no artificial flavors or dyes.

The food industry is masterful at playing on the stresses of modern parenthood. Its marketing people know that moms like Dana make the vast majority of household purchasing decisions, collectively spending more than two trillion dollars a year.[1] Food companies market to a population of parents they see as overwhelmed, harried, and racked with guilt and doubt. Dana's negative feelings are all "pain points" that the industry tries to "solve" by pushing its products. It delivers these solutions by bombarding parents with convenient processed products that let the parents supposedly have it all: they can both please their kids and ease their own guilty consciences. Companies promote the idea that kids don't like adult food and that their products offer healthy, child-friendly alternatives. They package their products tastefully, evoking a sense of health and naturalness while making false or meaningless health claims ("calcium-rich," "30 percent less sodium," "gluten-free," "with probiotics"). They sneak language referring to fruits and vegetables into their packaging, even if those ingredients are minimal additions to the products. Kix cereal's "Kid-Tested, Parent-Approved" slogan underscores the message that kids should pick their foods and then parents should approve, not the other way around.[2]

All of these ploys work.

"'Real cinnamon'?" Dana read on the box of Cinnamon Toast Crunch Paige handed to her. "How about Cheerios?" she asked Paige, who was staring up at her mom expectantly. Paige shook her head adamantly and glared in my direction, perhaps to enlist me as an advocate on her behalf. Dana rolled her eyes and looked down at the box in her hands. Here, too, whole grains were listed as the first ingredient. "Well," Dana said with a sigh, tossing the carton into the shopping cart, "how bad can they be?"

Madison and Paige weren't the only kids nagging their mom for foods filled with sugar, salt, and fat. Moms across the income spectrum experienced the same onslaught of requests from their kids. I witnessed this during shopping trips with Nyah, Renata, and the other parents I interviewed for my research. Not one mom completely escaped Big Food's aggressive marketing or their kids' desires for Cap'n Crunch or Chips Ahoy. Not one mom left the supermarket without making an unwanted compromise to appease her child. Not one mom felt great about everything listed on her grocery receipt.

"They always want junk," Julie Cain told me one afternoon as we prepared a pot of beef chili for dinner. "I mean, they really ask for a lot of it." Whenever Julie announced that she was going to Trader Joe's, Jane and Evan reliably had requests. Chips, cookies, soda—you name it, they wanted it.

Jane and Evan loved swinging by Starbucks after school to get Frappuccinos and going to Jamba Juice on the weekends for peanut butter–chocolate smoothies. When they went to the movies, they wanted buttered popcorn. When they went to the mall, they asked for slices of pizza. These foods brought genuine smiles to their faces.

In general, I saw Dana, Nyah, and moms with similar resources saying yes to their kids' requests. I also saw them occasionally say no. Nyah drew the line one evening after Natasha had eaten too many bags of Cheetos. Dana wouldn't let Paige get Starbucks after six o'clock because she didn't want her having that much caffeine and sugar before bed. But most often, lower-income moms' refusals derived from financial necessity; they largely said no to their kids when they didn't have the money. When discretionary funds were there, these moms strove to oblige.

Moms like Nyah and Dana said yes to junk food as a means

of buffering their kids against hardship. In saying yes and honoring their children's food requests, moms showed their kids that they saw them, that they heard them, and that they could give them not just what they *needed* but also what they *wanted*. Honoring and nurturing kids also meant giving them choices. In a context where moms felt like they didn't have all the options to present to their kids, that their kids' lives were already constrained by the realities of growing up in poverty, food was one of the few things kids really got to choose. Life was hard enough, and to take that agency away—to tell their kids they were wrong to want and ask for small indulgences—felt almost cruel.

"It makes them happy," Nyah had told me about junk food one afternoon as we pulled the car into the driveway. This rang true to me. Mariah and Natasha asked for treats like Pop-Tarts and Kool-Aid all the time and were elated when their mom obliged. When her mom handed her money for fast food, Mariah did a little dance—complete with a two-step and head nod—that made all of us erupt in laughter.

By contrast, I generally saw higher-income moms like Julie defaulting to no to these requests. The same was true, though to a slightly lesser degree, for Renata; even though Renata obliged her kids' requests more often than Julie, her general inclination was to say no rather than yes to their asks for Cheetos and Mars bars.

One evening, Julie and I stood in the kitchen making pasta. Dropping the long strands of spaghetti into a boiling pot of water, she recounted the fights that she'd gotten into with Jane and Evan. "Apparently I don't buy enough junk food." She chuckled, giving the dancing noodles a stir. "They say, 'I don't ever have things in my lunch box. You don't buy enough treats,'" Julie said, imitating her nagging kids. "But I just am pretty much like, 'No, no, and no.'"

Actually, Julie didn't *always* say no. She and Renata chose their battles. Sometimes, Julie was too exhausted to fight. She got tired of hearing Jane and Evan complain about not getting enough of the foods they asked for, and Jane and Evan similarly grew frustrated at their mom when she too quickly dismissed their requests. The kids also knew how to push their mom's buttons. For instance, Jane would turn Julie's and Zach's consumption of Diet Coke against them—if her parents could have soda, why couldn't she? Sometimes, Julie found herself at her wit's end. In those moments, she took the path of least resistance and indulged her kids.

Still, Julie and other affluent mothers maintained the general approach of saying no. This was in part motivated by a shared desire to keep kids' diets healthy. But I also saw that Julie's parenting context uniquely shaped what saying no meant to her and also how saying no *felt* to her. Saying no to the big stuff wasn't something that Julie had to navigate. Her ability to say yes to more of her children's needs and wants translated directly into an abundance of daily opportunities, big and small, for Julie to show her kids that she loved and cared for them. She gave them summer camps, weekend tutoring, and new laptops. She took them shopping, toured private high schools with Jane, and visited colleges with Evan. Food was neither a unique thing she could offer her kids nor a rare gift she could say yes to, so Julie didn't have to use food as a daily buffer against hardship. Food didn't serve the same purpose for Julie as it did for Nyah.

Julie's context also meant that saying no to junk food wasn't as emotionally distressing to her as a mother. What was one no in light of a thousand yeses? When Julie said no to Jane's pleas for salt and vinegar chips, she didn't worry about whether she was potentially harming or depriving her daughter.

Like Nyah and Dana, Julie and Renata used food to provide their kids with love and care, to nourish and sustain them. But each mom's broader parenting context changed *how* she used food to accomplish that goal.

Saying yes and saying no was as much about the moms as it was about the kids. Moms used food to care for their children, but they also used food for themselves—to feel a sense of worth as caregivers. Food wasn't just about kids' well-being; it was about moms' too. The food industry knows that. That's why it preys on moms so intensely, taunting them with that generally elusive prize of satisfying kids while also feeling like good caregivers.

But what does it mean to be a "good" mom? What were Julie, Dana, Renata, and Nyah all striving for in the first place?

In the United States, we share deeply held beliefs about what makes women good mothers. Sociologists refer to these beliefs as "the ideology of intensive mothering." The sociologist Sharon Hays coined the term *intensive mothering* in 1996 when she detailed the unreasonable, gendered demands society had increasingly placed on mothers since the 1980s. In the 1980s and 1990s, as more women in North America became educated and began entering the labor force, the intensive-mothering ideology arose as a means to redomesticate women through motherhood. The ideology specifies that good moms must act as kids' primary caregivers. Good mothering is child-centered and labor-intensive; good moms devote all of their energy, emotion, and attention to their kids. Good moms also listen to experts (for example, doctors and public health officials) to protect kids from harm and pave their way to success. Good moms are self-sacrificing; they put kids' needs before their own and forgo whatever is necessary—time, money, one's own dinner or mental health—to ensure their kids' well-being and happiness.[3] In a country with few legal protections and supportive policies for mothers, such as legally mandated paid maternity leave and universal childcare, intensive-mothering ideals have vested children's well-being almost exclusively in moms' hands.[4]

This notion that raising kids is a highly individual rather than communal or societal endeavor also favors more privileged, resourced moms who are less reliant on the state. That means that good moms in America end up being seen as white, married to men, monogamous, and stay-at-home caregivers. Because of this, being a good mom in the United States is an exclusionary ideal, challenging for all, attainable by few, and demanding of the highest level of selflessness and devotion.

Intensive mothering's standards are both unachievable and deeply gendered. The ideology dictates that mothers should not need or want the help of others—for instance, fathers and partners—in raising children. It specifies that mothers should also gladly engage in self-sacrifice in the name of their kids' best interests. It devalues mothers' inherent worth as humans, shifting that worth to how well they enact the role of their children's caretakers. It vests moms' dignity in motherhood, making children the metric by which society evaluates them and by which they come to value themselves. Intensive mothering dooms moms to feelings of inadequacy and the sense that they never do enough—that they never *are* enough.

Despite the ideology's unreasonable and unachievable standards, sociologists have found that moms across society buy into it. Although many recognize—and even critique—the level of stringency and self-sacrifice intensive mothering requires, they still feel beholden to its ideals and want to live up to them.[5] Put simply, moms across society aspire to be intensive mothers.

Intensive mothering has everything to do with what food means to moms. For one, feeding children is broadly considered to be mothers' inherent, biologically dictated responsibility. It starts with pregnancy, when most moms grow and develop their children in utero. It continues with breastfeeding, when moms are again expected to use their own bodies to fuel their children. While the physiological component disappears after that stage, moms continue to be viewed as naturally best poised to nourish and sustain their children. This powerful sentiment is held across society, within families, and often by moms themselves. It helps drive the reality in today's society that feeding is almost always the moms' primary responsibility.[6]

Food's centrality to motherhood made it a fitting, ongoing tool for the moms I met to enact intensive mothering. Food was an avenue for moms to devote resources, sacrifice their own needs or wants, and ensure their kids' well-being. It was a metric by which moms felt accountable and judged. Food was how moms strove to live up to intensive mothering's ideals. It was how they tried to stand tall and say, loud and clear, *I'm a good mom.*

But the very different worlds in which the moms I observed were raising their kids drove how specifically they used food to accomplish this goal of being "good." Saying yes to junk-food requests was how low-income moms worked to prove to themselves they were good mothers; saying no was how affluent moms tried to derive that exact same sense of worth.

I thought back to my evening at Target with Dana. Dana had let Madison and Paige fill the shopping cart with frozen pizzas and sugary yogurts, forgoing the bags of grapes and bunches of bananas she'd been eyeing. Obliging Madison's pleas for Dr Pepper and Paige's squeals for Rice Krispies Treats was to some degree about keeping the peace; Dana would do anything to avoid a battle with the girls at the end of a long day. She also wanted to make sure Madison and Paige felt provided for.

But there was more to it than that. Letting the girls grab whatever they wanted off the shelves was intimately tied to Dana's desire to feel competent in a world that too often told her she wasn't. While Dana didn't want her kids eating junk, she also couldn't bear to hear herself say no to one more of their asks. It would remind her of how limited she was, of how many noes she'd said so far in their lives and how many more she'd have to say. Good moms, Dana believed, had more to give their kids. Good moms found a way to say yes when it mattered.

So, staring at a six-pack of soda Paige had placed in the shopping cart, Dana nodded. "That's fine," she said with a sigh, rounding the corner into the freezer section.

I saw the same thing when I watched Nyah say yes to her

daughters. Junk food was certainly a gift to her kids, a momentary satisfaction of their dietary wants and the reason for Mariah's hilarious dance. But saying yes gave Nyah something too. As a Black, single, low-income mom, Nyah never felt like she could do enough—like she *was* enough. Whether in her daughters' pediatrician's office or during a meeting with her social worker, Nyah got the message loud and clear, every single day, that she did not fit society's definition of a good mom. The possibility of proving that wrong could seem futile. Nyah navigated stigma and judgment simply for existing and raising her kids as the woman she was. But the daily act of saying yes and bringing smiles to her daughters' faces offered Nyah a rare, welcome glimmer of hope. It suggested to her that maybe she was a better, more competent mother than the world cast her as.

In contrast, Julie and other affluent moms seemed to derive feelings of gratification by doing the exact opposite when it came to junk food. Julie sometimes laughed when she told me about denying her kids' requests. Certainly, in the moment, the requests annoyed and even wore her out. But it struck me that Julie was, at least in hindsight, proud about every time she was able to say no. She seemed, almost, to *enjoy* it. And that enjoyment, I realized, stemmed from how saying no made Julie feel.

Julie didn't face the same kind of societal scrutiny as Dana and Nyah about whether she was a good mom. According to the dogma of intensive mothering, she was. She was white. She was married. She was affluent. She was the definition of a child-centered caregiver, having chosen to prioritize raising her children over pursuing a professional path. She was equipped with resources to enact intensive mothering: more money in the bank, more space to move in, more gas in her car, more time to rest. Unlike Nyah and Dana, she was rarely asked to justify her parenting—no one asked Julie to defend buying her kids iPhones and expensive clothes. Society trusted Julie as a mother, a trust it did not bestow on those with less economic or racial

privilege. If any mom was poised to achieve intensive mothering's standards, it was Julie.

And yet just because Julie fit the definition didn't mean that
she always felt like a good mom. Even Julie, with all the resources
in the world, sometimes felt like she wasn't doing enough. Like
she could be working harder. Like she could be doing better.
Like she could *be* better.

It was this gnawing feeling of inadequacy—that little voice
in the back of every mom's head that told her she was falling
short—that kept Julie and other affluent moms continually trying to find ways to invest more energy, time, and money in their
children. Food offered an opportune outlet to channel these
efforts. Not only were moms held accountable and harshly
judged for their kids' intake and bodies, but food was also omnipresent. Keeping their kids' food nutritious and curbing kids'
unhealthy preferences were things affluent moms could work
on every single day and, in doing so, try to meet the bar of intensive mothering.

Simply put, saying no reflected Julie's deep commitment to
intensive mothering. Julie demonstrated her devotion to her
kids' nutritional well-being by continually striving to stem their
unhealthy cravings. Sure, it could be exhausting and frustrating
or even devolve into a battle. But Julie's willingness to wage a
yearslong war against her kids' desire for sugary and salty snacks
proved to her that she was willing to do anything that was in her
kids' best interests, even if they didn't see it that way. That's why
Julie said no. That's why Julie beamed with pride when she
talked about how frustrated her kids were that she never bought
"fun stuff." Julie beamed because, with every denial of her kids'
unhealthy requests, she found momentary proof that she was a
good mom.

CHAPTER 8

Hunger and Pickiness

For low-income moms, financial scarcity could give way to food scarcity. The ever-present threat of running out of money meant living with the fear that food could also just as easily run out.

Such fears were often rooted in moms' prior experiences. Nyah, for instance, knew what it was like not to have enough to fill her daughters' stomachs. The memory that haunted her most viscerally came from a time when Mariah was still in diapers. One evening, the six-month-old had awoken from a nap and proceeded to drink all of the formula intended to last two more days. With the formula depleted and no money to immediately restock it, Nyah paid her local food pantry a visit. There, she learned that they wouldn't be getting any formula in for another twenty-four hours. Desperate, Nyah returned home and tried giving her daughter whole milk. But the taste was foreign and unappetizing; Mariah spit it out and wailed from hunger. Nyah called her aunt who lived an hour away, and she promised to bring Nyah some more formula the next morning. Nyah stayed up all night with crying Mariah while she awaited her aunt. Sixteen years later, when Nyah closed her eyes, she could still hear her ravenous daughter's screams. Nyah never wanted her daughter to be in that kind of pain again—and she'd do everything in her power to make sure she never was.

Nyah wasn't alone. Other low-income moms had similar stories to share—some distant memories like Nyah's and others more recent. But whenever they had transpired, these prior experiences of food scarcity were seared into moms' brains. And the constant fear that such an experience could recur without warning shaped moms' priorities when it came to feeding kids. That is, the looming threat of food scarcity made their kids' current satiety a top priority for mothers.

Delfina Carrillo, a spunky single mom of three and a supermarket cashier, exemplified this prioritization. I met Delfina one afternoon in the three-bedroom, twelve-hundred-square-foot apartment she shared with her youngest son, fifteen-year-old Luis. Delfina, a second-generation Mexican-American, wore a blue tank top and jean shorts that hit right above her knee. Chatty and candid, Delfina paired a contagious laugh with a tendency to gesture enthusiastically.

Like Nyah, Delfina had lived through periods when the fridge was empty and the freezer was headed in that direction too. Feeding herself and her three kids on a cashier's salary had been a feat of magic that she'd worked hard to pull off, all while trying to hide the emotional toll that struggle took. For years, what had proven extremely stressful for Delfina was that all three of her children—who loved sports and seemed to rotate through growth spurts on a weekly basis—were always hungry.

"They had serious appetites." Delfina chuckled, rubbing her stomach.

Some afternoons, the kids returned home from school insatiable. And if money hadn't been an issue for Delfina, her kids' appetites wouldn't have been either. If they'd wanted second or third helpings of dinner every night, she could easily have bought more food.

But money was an issue, and therefore, so was their hunger. While two of her three children were now grown and living outside her home, Delfina would never forget the lesson she'd learned over the years of filling their bellies. That lesson was that she had to be painstakingly intentional about how she grocery shopped—about how and where she put her hard-earned dollars toward food. If Delfina wasn't careful, she could easily blow through the week's earnings on food that didn't fill her kids up and left them tossing and turning in their beds from growling stomachs. Delfina learned to prioritize satiety.

But another hard lesson that Delfina learned was that her kids could be as picky as they were ravenous. This is a lesson many parents learn at some point, and often the hard way. They discover that trying to get toddlers and children to eat something new comes with risks. Giving kids unfamiliar and less preferred foods can lead to battles, ones that kids are more likely than parents to win. When her kids were little, Delfina discovered that even if her children were starving, they wouldn't eat just anything. They could—and often did—turn down dishes they didn't like, even throwing them onto the floor. When this happened, Delfina grew frustrated and more stressed: not only was that food on the floor wasted, but Delfina was out the money that it had cost her to buy it.

The sociologist Caitlin Daniel has written about the bind that kids' pickiness creates for low-income moms. Daniel interviewed moms of young children and observed their trips to the supermarket, and she discovered that low-income moms had to consider not only how much food cost but also what would happen if their kids refused it. "To avoid risking waste," Daniel explained in her *New York Times* opinion piece, "these parents fall back on their children's preferences."[1]

The low-income moms I met faced the same food-waste concerns and responded similarly. The moms explained that they'd learned early on in their kids' lives that catering to kids' preferences was a more financially sound choice than attempting to force new foods on them. Catering to what children wanted all but eliminated the possibility of wasted food and money. When moms customized shopping lists to kids' tastes, then whatever food they bought was consumed and contributed to their children's growth and satiety.

Delfina's drive to fill Luis up at home was related to the fact that Luis often went hungry during the day. Delfina worried because Luis, like Ebony—the vegan teenager from chapter 4—frequently skipped school lunch. Having eaten it since elementary school, he had grown tired of the monotony of flavors and textures. What was on offer never seemed to change. Sometimes, to tide himself over until school let out, Luis turned to the school snack shop. There, he'd buy Smart Snacks.

Since 2014, the food industry has reformulated popular brands of snacks to meet the CDC's Smart Snacks in Schools standards but packaged them to resemble the widely available, less nutritious versions. These look-alike versions of junk food get kids exposed and hooked. Luis could buy reduced-fat or low-sodium versions of his favorite snacks, like Cheetos, Doritos, and Sour Worms. The packaging was the same, the taste virtually identical, and the price under two dollars a bag.[2] Outside of school, when they stopped at a gas station or picked up school supplies from Walmart, Luis would ask his mom for those same treats. Delfina would oblige, unaware that his school was helping cultivate her son's demand for the junk she wished he'd avoid.

But when Luis didn't have the money to buy school snacks, he returned home in the early afternoon starving and ready to raid the family's kitchen.[3] Those afternoons, Delfina catered to Luis's requests because doing so ensured he wouldn't go hungry. She got him what he asked for. Sometimes that involved buying him Papa John's, Taco Bell, or Panda Express. Other times, it meant that Delfina cooked for Luis. She asked him before going to the supermarket exactly what he wanted so she could be sure to purchase something he'd eat. Delfina knew that if she bought or baked Luis a pizza, he would definitely fill up on it. But if she insisted that he eat green beans, he might go to bed hungry.

"The most important thing to me is that I have something Luis likes so he will eat," Delfina said, running a hand through her thick brown hair. "He's happy. I'm happy."

Indeed, when Delfina plopped down with Luis on the couch after a long day, she was quick to sacrifice her own food preferences to assure her son's. She'd get Luis whatever he wanted and try to fill herself up with something shelf-stable. It was not unusual for Delfina to skip a meal so Luis could order Domino's. Delfina would grab something off the shelf of soups, beans, and flour tortillas she kept in the kitchen cupboard for exactly that reason. The stuff she got from the food pantry wasn't her favorite, but it was edible. Delfina sometimes ate less so that Luis could eat more. Delfina went to bed hungry so Luis wouldn't have to.

This is the irony of many moms who work in the food system—in supermarkets, like Delfina, at restaurants, or on farms. Surrounded by food all day, they find themselves food-insecure and constantly worried about their children's satiety. Indeed, food workers in the U.S. are more likely to experience food insecurity than workers in other industries. The numbers are even starker for restaurant employees, who report food insecurity at double the rate of the U.S. population. And compared to their male and white counterparts, women and workers of color like Delfina are more likely to be food-insecure.[4] Delfina helped make the food system run, but she couldn't afford to reliably feed herself or her kids the way she wanted.

Thinking about what to eat for dinner that night, Delfina told me she'd probably order Luis a pizza. She grimaced, joking about how sick she was of cheese and bread. But then, leaning back on the couch, Delfina grinned. "As long as he eats," she said, shrugging, "I'm happy."

While moms like Delfina were focused on ensuring their kids had *enough* to eat, wealthier moms often seemed more concerned about their kids having *too much* to eat—especially of the "wrong" things. That ability to worry about the particulars of kids' diets, I came to see, was an inequitably distributed luxury. Knowing that there would be enough to fill their children's bellies, wealthier moms focused on the details of what went into those bellies. Rather than losing sleep over whether the foods their kids ate were satiating, moms instead focused on sculpting kids' preferences.

"We don't eat for comfort," Julie explained to me one afternoon while we sat on the couch watching TV, folding laundry, and awaiting Jane's return from school. I asked Julie if she talked to her kids about that. Did her kids know that they shouldn't be eating for comfort? Of course, Julie replied, flipping through the channels, landing ultimately on CNN. But it wasn't like she wanted them *not* to enjoy food. Rather, Julie said, she wanted Evan and Jane to love food but also know that its primary purpose was to keep them alive.

"I also want them to think, *Well, I don't necessarily need all this food either,*" Julie clarified. "*My body can do without it.*"

Julie's comment about restricting certain foods reminded me of Patricia Adams, a white single mom with an easy laugh and an eye for order. I joined Patricia's family at home on a calm winter evening, and the two of us sat kitty-corner at a kitchen table with bright yellow checkered place mats and a vase of pink tulips in the center. Patricia, who had a master's degree in education and worked as a private-school teacher, had just finished cleaning up from dinner. Her eldest daughter, Zoe, was on her way home from volleyball practice, and her two younger daughters, Mary and Louise, were finishing up their homework in the living room. Every occasion that Patricia and her daughters were around food, she told me, presented an opportunity for her to teach them something about what to eat and what not to eat.

"I've done my own bit of research on food," Patricia told me, straightening out the place mat. "So I try to buy organic and healthy and limit the amount of fat and hydrogenated oils that we eat. It's really important to me what we eat."

Despite the fact that Patricia and Delfina were both single

moms working full-time with kids at home, their situations diverged sharply. Compared to Delfina's job as a cashier, Patricia's job as a teacher paid significantly more and came with benefits that gave her retirement savings and health insurance. Her work hours allowed her to drop the kids off at school and be home prepping dinner before they returned. While she too was on her feet much of the day, she never worked nights or weekends. She never had her hours cut or her wages stolen. Patricia received child support from her ex-husband. She had more time to spend with her kids and more money to make use of that time the way she wanted than Delfina had.

Patricia's resources meant she didn't have to worry about her kids' hunger the way Delfina did. That her kids would be full was a given. Indeed, never once did Patricia mention her children's hunger or satiety as relevant concerns. Patricia's resources also meant that she didn't need to worry about the financial implications of wasted food. She didn't love throwing food away, but if her daughters didn't want to eat their broccoli, there were no serious economic consequences. Because of this, Patricia did not need to cater to her daughters' preferences. Patricia's financial security allowed her to turn any signs of her kids' pickiness into what she called "teaching moments."

"As a parent, everything you do is a teaching moment," she told me, rolling up the sleeves of her flannel shirt and leaning forward to rest her elbows on the table.

Night after night, Patricia could put stalks of broccoli on her kids' plates. It didn't matter if her kids refused once, twice, or fifteen times. It didn't matter if they tossed that broccoli into the trash can or onto the kitchen tiles. Patricia had the financial reserves to buy more. Running out of food or money was not an issue. Her kids' pickiness, from a financial perspective, was irrelevant. It didn't factor into her food purchases, and it didn't stop her from trying to convince them — for the hundredth time — to eat their vegetables.

Teaching moments abounded in Patricia's world. Whether it was how to read a nutrition label, scramble an egg, or exercise portion control, Patricia was always thinking about what lessons she could instill in her girls. She wanted to show them how to exercise self-restraint and control around food. She tried to teach them how to develop "better" tastes and overcome what she saw as inferior ones.

I thought of Delfina when Patricia started talking to me about salty snacks. Like Luis, Patricia's daughters had come across Smart Snacks in school. They'd seen their friends buy the food industry's school-approved potato chips and candy bars. And they'd come home to tell their mom that they wanted to eat Cheez-Its and Goldfish just like their classmates.

"I'm like, 'Oh my God, I don't want to give my kids fishy crackers!'" Patricia exclaimed, remembering her horror at her kids' request. "Especially not the red, blue, or green ones or whatever those are."

Patricia didn't want her girls ingesting food coloring and additives. She couldn't bear the idea of that stuff making its way into their bodies. Patricia believed, as many affluent moms I spoke to did, in the importance of raising what the sociologists Kate Cairns, Josée Johnston, and Norah MacKendrick call the "organic child." Raising an organic child means more than getting your kid to eat vegetables and fruits, although that's essential. It also goes beyond choosing organic over conventional produce. Raising an organic kid is about so much more. It means making carefully calculated, informed, and often costly decisions about what goes into your child's body. It means making baby food by hand, reading the fine print on labels, researching omega-3 to omega-6 ratios, and thinking about the plastic packaging encasing granola bars and milk cartons.[5]

The ideal of feeding kids an organic diet has, over the past decade, become a kind of gold standard of healthy child-rearing. This standard is generally communicated to and absorbed by moms across society, although it's largely accomplished in full by only the most privileged. That is, it's a feature of intensive mothering reserved almost exclusively for moms like Patricia and Julie. News media and public health initiatives target these moms to tell them it is their responsibility to protect their kids from an unsafe, risky, and contaminated food industry that puts artificial dye in crackers, infuses arsenic into baby food, and keeps kids' palates from developing by packing children's menus with cheeseburgers and French fries. Interestingly, moms today get the message that it is their job to safeguard their kids, not that it's the state's responsibility to regulate and monitor industry practices.

The organic-child ideal creates yet another hoop for "good" moms to jump through and a set of impossible standards that even the most privileged caregivers, like Patricia, feel they are at constant risk of falling short of. Patricia was always looking for ways to keep her growing girls in an organic bubble. She tried to find a healthier alternative to the conventional Cheez-Its, one that she could live with as a mom without depriving her kids. She researched online and in-store at Whole Foods. She read labels. She talked to her friends. Finally, she found a substitute that, although pricey, met the minimum criteria for her: Annie's Cheddar Squares.

"It had natural coloring, organic cheddar, no hydrogenated oil," Patricia said, breathing a sigh of relief. For that moment, Patricia felt good about how she had handled the Cheez-It dilemma. She had neither given in nor given up. She had transformed an unhealthy preference into a teaching moment.

Patricia worked hard to keep her home an organic bubble, safe from the food industry. She also saw her teaching moments paying off more and more. Sure, her kids still asked for things like Cheez-Its and Oreos. And yes, they still ordered pizza with their friends and got buttered popcorn at the movies. This was inevitable. But Patricia could tell that they now had an ingrained taste for nutritious foods like quinoa, salads, squash, and cashews. Rather than succumbing to her kids' pickiness, she had flipped the script—*she* was making *them* picky for the right foods.

One of Patricia's proudest moments happened when, as a last resort on a road trip, she swung by Taco Bell with her daughters. It was late, they were in the middle of nowhere, and everyone was hungry. Patricia acted out of desperation but worried that she would later pay the consequences of that decision. What if her girls loved fast food? What if they started asking for it nonstop? What if all of her years of hard work were undone with one bite?

"But," Patricia said cheerfully as she told me the story, "they didn't like the bean burrito! They didn't like the taste. Not at all!" Patricia beamed at the memory of her kids actively rejecting fast food, registering it as proof of her own success. She recalled with pride how they'd tossed their half-eaten burritos in the parking lot's trash can before getting back in the car.

As Patricia recounted her success story, I thought of Delfina. I thought of how differently this story would have played for Delfina—how bad she would have felt if Luis had wasted half his dinner. I thought of the frustration it would have caused her to see her son discard perfectly edible, satiating food that she'd worked hard to be able to buy. I thought of the financial stress she would have endured as she wondered whether she had enough money to get him something else. I thought about how Patricia's proudest teaching moment was Delfina's nightmare.

CHAPTER 9

Status Symbols

Sometimes I wondered if food's nutritional content was all that moms like Patricia cared about. Certainly, their desire to keep their kids healthy and protected from the food system was part of the story. But it wasn't the whole story.

Moms like Patricia also cared about food as a signifier of their social position—a status symbol. If we are what we eat, then the food we put in our bodies says as much about our identities and location in the social hierarchy as it does about our health. The moms I met cared about food's reputation, about what eating certain ingredients and buying particular brands signaled to the world about who they were as individuals as well as what kind of parents they were. They cared about who else consumed those foods and bought those brands. These criteria, which sometimes had very little to do with food's nutritional properties, helped moms decide whether something was appropriate for their children to eat.

Patricia's Cheez-It substitution reflected these considerations. Patricia's concern about her daughters' health motivated her to search for an alternative cracker. But it wasn't clear how much more nutritious Annie's Cheddar Squares were. Calorically, the two items were nearly identical: 150 calories for twenty-seven Cheez-Its and 140 for the same number of cheddar squares. The former had 8 grams of fat, 1.5 grams of which were saturated fat; the latter had 7 grams of fat, 1 gram of which was saturated fat. Interestingly, a serving of Cheez-Its contained 20 milligrams *less* sodium than cheddar squares did. Each cracker had a lengthy list of ingredients, but the cheddar square had organic ones and did not contain the hydrogenated oils in Cheez-Its.

Overall, the cheddar squares were probably slightly healthier than the Cheez-Its. But neither snack was an apple. And yet Patricia felt so strongly about her daughters consuming the organic version over the conventional one. And she was not alone. Moms labeled certain products as unacceptable while being okay with others that were nutritionally comparable. They derided Cheetos but let their kids eat Barbara's Cheese Puffs. They pointed out that they never ate McDonald's, but they regularly visited In-N-Out Burger as a family. A bean burrito from Taco Bell was unacceptable but getting the exact same thing from a local taqueria made them culturally open-minded and cosmopolitan. Julie, for instance, wholeheartedly approved of Trader Joe's Joe-Joe's cookies but discouraged her children from eating nearly identical Oreos. One mom told me that Friday nights were pizza nights at her house, but she always made sure to order a "good pizza" and not "the five-dollar pizza," which she saw as devoid of any nutrition.

But what was the difference between a Joe-Joe and an Oreo? What distinguished a good pizza from a bad one? What made a food acceptable or unacceptable?

Often, the label—and its associations—mattered most. It mattered that Julie's Joe-Joe's could be purchased only at Trader Joe's and couldn't be found in any old gas station. It mattered that the pizza was prepared by a local restaurant and not a national chain. It mattered how moms answered this question: Do people like us eat this?

Do people like us cruise through Burger King drive-throughs?

Do people like us frequent all-you-can-eat buffets?

Do people like us have Froot Loops for breakfast?

Do people like us shop at the dollar store?

If the answer was no, then that food was not an acceptable choice.

By "people like us," moms generally meant people who looked like them — the ones they saw around them on neighborhood sidewalks and in school parking lots. Most of the moms I interviewed, like many Americans, lived in sharply segregated neighborhoods. Their children attended schools with relatively homogenous student populations. There were exceptions, of course. But often, those closest to the families I interviewed resembled them racially and socioeconomically. And moms' ideas about how these proximate, similar others ate informed their understanding of what was an appropriate diet.

Such ideas also influenced where families shopped for groceries. Store prices and proximity were certainly part of the calculus. But so too was whether a store felt right or wrong, whether moms saw themselves reflected in the clientele or noticed cars like theirs in the parking lot. That was one reason why Patricia loved Whole Foods and Julie Trader Joe's, why Dana shopped at Target and Nyah Grocery Outlet. These were the places where they felt at home. These were the supermarkets where they felt like they belonged.

But there was a flip side to wealthier moms' food purchases. On the one hand, they bought organic versions of popular products and frequented "higher-quality" fast-food establishments. These choices communicated moms' elevated tastes. But many of these moms also went to great lengths to show me that their tastes weren't *too* elevated or highbrow. They weren't overbearing, extremist health freaks who deprived their children of all salt, sugar, and fat. They weren't pretentious snobs. They too shared an appreciation of less healthy, less "sophisticated" foods.

Often, moms showcased their humility and easygoingness to me by zeroing in on one or two products that they felt made them seem down-to-earth. One mom discussed her love of Eggo waffles and her disdain of Whole Foods' whole-wheat, gluten-free substitutes. Another noted that her kids ate only McDonald's fries, which were cut and salted to perfection; oven-baked sweet potato wedges could never compare. One emphasized that she bought her kids the classic Fig Newtons rather than the dense, organic fig bars she found in the supermarket bulk section. And another told me that she would *never* make her son a grilled cheese with anything but the "super-processed Kraft slices" of American cheese; well-aged Brie or goat cheese was delicious but completely inappropriate.

I believed moms, but I also suspected they were making a big deal out of their "humbler" tastes to dispel any notion I might have of them as elitist. I wondered if they mentioned these foods in order to downplay their privilege.

If that was the case, then these efforts only underscored their privilege to me. When it suited them, these moms could glorify feeding their kids less nutritious foods in a way that less privileged moms couldn't without being criticized. The former used these foods to show that they were grounded, reasonable caregivers—good moms who practiced moderation and didn't go to extremes. Sometimes, these moms were saying, they could be laid-back, or even fun! Offering Kraft American cheese and Fig Newtons as evidence of good parenting was a luxury that lower-income moms didn't have. Were these moms to talk openly about feeding their kids those products, they would be regarded as negligent for not caring enough or lazy for choosing shortcuts that undermined their kids' health. They would be deemed "bad" moms even if they were serving their kids the same foods the "good" moms were. When privileged and less privileged moms fed their kids the exact same thing, I learned, the former were viewed as down to earth while the latter were chastised for their choices.

Moms who had grown up poor but now identified as middle or upper middle class illustrated how clearly food operated as a status symbol. For these upwardly mobile moms, like Latisha Jenkins, their kids' diets were tangible evidence of their success in ascending the social hierarchy. Latisha helped me see how more privileged moms used their kids' diets to lay claim to their place in society. Food was about more than nourishment—it was about embodying and displaying a class identity.

Raised in Arizona in a small agricultural community, Latisha had moved to the Bay Area in the mid-1980s to attend Stanford. She had not planned to stay there, but after she met her husband and had children, it felt like home. Now a single mom of four, Latisha worked full-time at a local nonprofit. Latisha and I met late one afternoon in the Stanford student union. Her thick black hair pulled back tight in a low bun, Latisha had chestnut skin and carried a Harrods tote bag. Surrounded by students studying for midterms, we pulled up two plastic stools to a high communal table.

"It cracks me up to think that my kids will say they grew up in Palo Alto." Latisha laughed, looking around at hordes of students hunched over laptops. "But one day I guess they'll be able to say that!"

During her own childhood, Latisha never thought that much about food. Her mom put food on her plate, and she ate it. Latisha didn't remember ever being hungry, but she also didn't remember feeling excited about food. Eating was, as Latisha put it, instrumental. The fact that Latisha now had the resources to teach her kids about food and cultivate their palates was proof to her that she was doing better economically than her mother and father. The fact that she could choose between an Eggo and a Whole Foods waffle was a big deal.

"My lunches were terrible growing up," Latisha said, tucking a wiry strand of black hair behind her ear. "My lunches were Oscar Mayer deli meat in between two pieces of bread."

Thinking about the sandwiches she now sent her own kids to school with, Latisha continued, "It was never this lovely sandwich with lettuce and cheese and all these elements."

In college, Latisha started learning more about food—where it came from, how it tasted, what was healthy and what wasn't. These revelations fundamentally changed how Latisha thought about her own diet and, later, that of her kids. Latisha felt that her mom had thought comparatively little about food. Now Latisha took great pride in giving her kids what she called "better." She felt strongly about teaching her kids what she hadn't learned until her twenties. Her kids were growing up as part of the upper middle class, and she wanted them to act like it. They couldn't show up to private school with Oscar Mayer deli meat. She wanted them to love avocados and rustic loaves of bread, heirloom tomatoes and poached eggs. Latisha had worked hard to get them to a higher rung of the class ladder. Now she wanted them to feel like they belonged there—and eat like it too. She also understood that her kids' peers and their families might make assumptions about her children's diets. She knew the racist stereotypes about how Black families like hers ate. She could imagine the jokes their classmates might make about her kids living on fried chicken and macaroni and cheese. She wanted to equip her kids to swiftly and seamlessly dismantle those misguided assumptions.

Because of this, Latisha took educating her kids about food seriously. Their futures, after all, depended on it. Like Patricia, Latisha was quick to identify teaching moments in daily life. Whether they were sitting down at a café or perusing the outer aisles of the supermarket, she always had something to show her children. At the farmers' market, Latisha said, "We smell things. We taste things. We look at how different things look." Latisha talked to her kids about what they were seeing. She made sure they knew what was right and what was wrong to eat.

Latisha wanted her kids to like certain foods, but she was

equally invested in making sure they didn't like—or even know about—certain foods that she had grown up with. Her family had come so far, and those foods could set them back.

"My kids don't eat bad lunch meat." Latisha smiled. "They only have kosher, wonderful, flavored salamis and all these kinds of things. Great cheeses. Not just some processed cheese. They know different cheeses. They know how different cheeses taste." Latisha felt proud that they ate only Fuji and Pink Lady apples. "They couldn't imagine eating a mushy, tasteless, thick-skinned apple," she said, beaming. They were similarly clueless about products like bologna, Ding-Dongs, and Twinkies.

"What's a Twinkie?" Latisha's daughter had asked her mom one afternoon after seeing it at a friend's house. Latisha explained that they didn't eat Twinkies.

"I'm like, 'We don't live like that.'" Latisha laughed, shifting in her seat. "'We don't *have* to live that way.'"

This, Latisha felt, was one of the greatest gifts she could give her kids. She could give them the luxury of choice. Taste and desire would drive their food selections, not necessity. And Latisha knew that eating well today would serve them well tomorrow. Latisha could see her kids' future now, and it excited her to envision her hard work paying off. One day, years from now, they would visit a law school professor's home for dinner or attend a networking function hosted by a prestigious firm. They would attend a wine-and-cheese function or be invited to a dinner at a fancy restaurant. Because they would know how to eat—and *enjoy*—the food on offer, her grown-up kids would thrive in those settings. Their elevated tastes would enable them to take advantage of the opportunities Latisha had worked hard to provide them. These tastes would allow them to achieve even greater social mobility than Latisha herself had. And these tastes would help solidify their place in the upper middle class, making it clear to anyone and everyone that they were there to stay.

CHAPTER 10

Kale Salad

There are many ways to eat nutritiously. And yet the media generally present a relatively narrow image of a healthy diet. They do this by drawing attention away from broad food groups and focusing on the merits and faults of specific foods or nutrients. Certain items are included in the "good" and "healthy" category while others are excluded and portrayed as "bad" and "unhealthy." These acts of inclusion and exclusion certainly have something to do with the foods' nutritional properties, but they also have a lot to do with these foods' cultural and racial associations and histories. Foods are classified as healthy not just because of what they are but also because of what they represent and who they have been historically produced and consumed by.

Discourses around soul food underscore this point. There's a reason why people sing the praises of kale but not collard greens. Throughout American history, in both the nutrition community and mass media, soul food has largely been derogated rather than celebrated. Although soul food is rooted in the historical and present-day resilience and survival of Black communities across America, it has generally been regarded as unhealthy, uncivilized, and backward. Foods that are culturally white—yogurt, cottage cheese, avocado toast, almonds, tofu, and salad—are paraded as healthy and sophisticated. Foods associated with Black culture—fried chicken, sweet potato pie, and biscuits—have consistently been stigmatized as inferior.[1]

Just as ideas about healthy foods are culturally and racially inculcated, so too are notions about *who* is healthy and what healthy *is*. For the most part, these associations unfairly position white families, white bodies, and white diets as healthier. Families of color—and bodies of color—are generally considered to be unhealthy, and their traditional diets are seen as deviant.[2]

Many of the moms of color I met were keenly aware of the racist narratives pervading dietary discourses. These moms wrestled with and fought against such narratives on a daily basis.

Janae Lathrop was one such mom. I met Janae on a balmy spring afternoon in the two-story home she shared with her husband, three daughters, and their fluffy, freckled Labradoodle. Janae had firsthand knowledge of the racist assumptions society made about how Black mothers fed themselves and their kids.

That knowledge, I came to understand, shaped our initial interactions. Janae had been challenging for me to schedule time with. Each time I had reached out to her over the previous few months, she was too busy to meet. I could see why; managing a job and a family of five made time a scarce resource. But when she and I finally connected, carving out a couple of hours on a Sunday afternoon, I realized that her hesitancy had had as much if not more to do with her concerns about me and my research as with scheduling constraints.

When I arrived, Janae opened the front door wearing a denim button-down collared shirt and pink workout leggings. She immediately invited me to take a tour of the first floor of her home. Walking through the bright entryway back into her chef's kitchen, I could see why she wanted to show it off. The kitchen was straight out of an interior-design magazine: Sunlight poured in through big windows onto a white, granite island. Atop the island were bowls of fresh fruit and a pristine

Vitamix blender. Cookbooks lined the built-in bookshelves above a silver gas stove.

"I didn't want to do anything formal when you came," Janae explained, casually pouring the smoothie she'd just made into two glasses and then passing one to me. "I just thought I could bring you into our life as it is."

Smoothies in hand, we migrated over to the living room to chat. Janae kicked her slippers off and curled her legs up on the couch as sunlight streamed in through the bay window. While Janae had told me up front that she'd budgeted only an hour for our conversation, that hour turned into two and a half once we eased into conversation. Janae was surprised that we were hitting it off. She made comments throughout the afternoon about how much fun our chat was turning out to be and how she wished she'd found the time earlier.

When I asked Janae to tell me about herself, she began by mentioning that she and her husband, Darryl, had advanced degrees—he an MBA from Harvard University, she a JD from the University of Massachusetts—and that, as two Black working professionals, she and Darryl were extremely active in giving back to low-income Black communities.

Then we started talking about food.

"Food for us was big growing up," Janae told me, bringing the smoothie to her lips and taking a quick sip. Janae's mother and grandmother were phenomenal cooks, preparing dishes not only for their families but also for weddings and church gatherings.

"You've heard of soul food?" She squinted at me optimistically.

"I have." I nodded, smiling.

"Good for you!" Janae exclaimed, setting the smoothie down on the glass coffee table. "My mother's specialties are soul food, so she cooks mostly casseroles and fish and baked chicken and greens—which is a big soul food—and black-eyed peas and corn bread and mac and cheese and yams. And she bakes. She makes red velvet cake. She makes peach cobbler. She makes pound cake and Seven-Up cake."

Janae paused, sitting up on the sofa.

"It's really different than how I cook," she said. "I'm more into organic and salads." Janae's mom didn't really get the way that Janae cooked for her family. That food was alien to her. Janae liked kale, Greek yogurt, and quinoa. "My mom doesn't do quinoa!" Janae laughed. "She does comfort food. I don't think she's even *said* quinoa before!"

Janae sprinkled comments like this throughout our conversation—comments that underscored how different she was from the rest of her extended family. These comments seemed slightly forced, motivated, perhaps, by a central thesis she wanted me to grasp. When she later mentioned that her parents always had chips at their house, she quickly added, "You're not gonna find any of that here!"

Janae saw her mom's cooking as partly the product of American racial segregation and discrimination. Her mom's opportunities had been limited and her exposure to other people and environments curtailed. "I mean, this is America, right?" Janae rolled her eyes. "We're talking demographics and who we are, and so as a culture, my mother and grandmother were only around mostly people just like them. That's how it was."

But things had been, in some ways, different for Janae, who had come of age in a later era. It was an era still characterized by widespread structural and institutional racism and unequal access to opportunities for Black communities, but Janae had more opportunities than any family members who had come before her. And she seized those opportunities with every fiber in her body, devoting herself to academics throughout her youth, proving wrong the teachers and college counselors who doubted or discouraged her, and ultimately landing a spot at a top university.

In college, Janae started learning about what went into her food. "I got exposed to new things and new cultures and new people and new experiences through my education," Janae said. "I was able to try other things, where for my mom and her mom, it was pretty limited." Janae started to question things she had once taken for granted. "That caused me to say, 'Oh, there might be more than just mac and cheese.'" Janae laughed. "Because mac and cheese is butter and cheese, and I know that that can't be all that healthy."

Janae committed herself to approaching food differently with her kids. Like Latisha, she attributed her new approach to her upward mobility. At the same time, Janae felt a deep attachment, warmth, and nostalgia for the food she'd been raised on. That was the food that had made her who she was today. So she tried to offer her daughters a bit of both worlds: the new stuff Janae was embracing plus the foods reflecting their culture and heritage.

"It's not all quinoa for my girls," Janae told me, placing her feet firmly on the floor and leaning forward. "I look to my mom too. Like, 'Mom, help me bring in some of that comfort food.'" She paused. "So I have my mom's influence, but then I'm bringing in all these other things that I was exposed to."

Janae was on my mind the next week when I met Harmony Ross, a nonprofit leader and mom of three. Janae and I had talked about one of her favorite foods, kale, and now the leafy green had come up with Harmony too.

Over the past decade, kale has been identified by elite foodies and restaurateurs as an "it" ingredient and deemed trendy as a healthy superfood. Health gurus tout the vegetable's nutritional punch. Restaurants feature kale salads with avocado dressing and bread crumbs. Supermarket aisles offer kale chips and kale flakes, and juice bars sell expensive kale smoothies for post–yoga workouts. Kale has become a status symbol; tote bags and sweatshirts feature phrases like EAT MORE KALE and OH KALE YES!

But while kale has surged in popularity, that popularity has been socioeconomically and racially skewed, as kale is generally marketed toward and endorsed by upper middle class, primarily white people. Because of that, while kale may be healthy, it is seen as a wealthy white person's food, making its appeal culturally limited and its glorification culturally alienating. While kale was attractive to Black moms like Janae because of their strong identification as high-income and well-educated members of society, some middle-class Black moms like Harmony were put off by it.

On a warm Wednesday afternoon, Harmony and I sat outside at a picnic bench. In black leggings and a gray track jacket, her brown hair pulled back in a high bun, Harmony looked like she was on her way to or from the gym. Her bright smile and resounding laugh matched her bright pink lipstick and diamond-studded bangles.

"My mother and father are from Georgia," Harmony told me. "So growing up, we had soul food—greens, cabbages, corn bread, potato salad, short ribs, starches, always dessert, sweet potato pie, cobbler, Seven-Up cake."

Harmony paused. "You know, just kind of soul food, Southern comfort food." When Harmony's family relocated from the South to the West Coast, her mom continued cooking those dishes, which were always eaten at lively and convivial family dinners.

Harmony mentioned kale a few times during our conversation, explaining that it was not a vegetable she would put in her shopping cart or one she'd order at a restaurant. To Harmony, kale was a skinny white woman's food—not hers. Harmony then told me a story about kale that she found so funny, she had trouble getting it out without erupting into laughter.

This was the story: Harmony's seventeen-year-old daughter,

Ida, recently visited a white friend's house after school. The two girls spent the afternoon hunched over the dining-room table solving calculus equations. When dinnertime rolled around, her friend's mom had offered to make them dinner.

"Guess what she made them?" Harmony asked me, her eyes widening and the sides of her mouth curling slightly upward.

"Something with kale?" I ventured. Harmony began vigorously nodding.

"She made them a kale salad!" She cackled, putting both hands on the table as if to brace herself. "Can you imagine?"

Harmony was tearing up from laughter. She called Ida, who was doing homework at a nearby table, over to join us.

"Ida," Harmony said to her daughter as she took a seat beside her mom on the bench, "what would you do if I made you a kale salad for dinner?"

Ida side-eyed her mom. "I would wonder where the meat is," she said, her tone deadpan.

They looked at each other and erupted in laughter.

Kale's whiteness and cultural otherness to Harmony and Ida had little, if anything, to do with the vegetable's nutritional properties or even its taste. Kale is, in fact, strikingly similar in flavor, texture, and nutrition to collard greens, which have long been a staple of traditional soul food and are still a mainstay in many Black households. Both Harmony and Nyah cooked collard greens every week, stewing the leaves in large frying pans with garlic and, sometimes, bits of bacon.

But it is no coincidence that kale, not collard greens, has been embraced by the healthy-eating community as a superfood.[3] And it is no surprise that some Black moms reject not only the vegetable but also mainstream healthy-eating recommendations advising them to eat "white people" foods like kale. Understandably, Harmony generally assumed those recommendations were from and for other people. Maybe Ida's white classmates, Harmony mused. But they certainly weren't meant for

her and her family because there was no way Harmony was tossing a bunch of shredded kale with balsamic vinaigrette, topping
it with pine nuts, and calling it dinner.

As Janae and I wrapped up our interview, we circled back to the
kitchen, where I rinsed my empty glass in the farmhouse sink.
Hesitantly, I asked Janae if she knew any other Black families
who might be willing to speak with me.

"Well, sure!" Janae answered eagerly, taking my glass and
putting it in the top rack of the dishwasher. Then she paused.
"What kind of Black families are you looking for?"

Janae said that she could point me toward the low-income
Black families from her church. "It's in the inner city," she said,
sighing. "Totally not like this neighborhood." I explained that at
this point in my research, I was actually hoping to speak with
other higher-income Black families like hers.

Janae looked genuinely surprised. Taken aback, even. "When
you wrote me," she said, "I was like, I might not be the African-
American family that she's looking for! Because most people
who interview African-American families—let's be real—they're
looking for this socioeconomic one that's the masses." Researchers, Janae said, didn't want to speak with Black people like her,
ones with law degrees and multimillion-dollar homes.

Janae's perception of the research community resonated
broadly with my own. With notable exceptions, social scientists
have had a long and problematic tradition of studying—focusing on, even—poor, urban communities of color. Because of
that, Janae had assumed I wanted to speak to a low-income
Black family. She was sure that I would be disappointed when I
met her and discovered that she wasn't the least bit poor.

That was why she'd put off the interview for so long. And
that was why, when we'd finally scheduled it, Janae had made it
very clear that her family was well-off, detailing how highly educated and high-earning she and her husband were. That's why

she'd made me that organic smoothie and offered me a tour of her kitchen and its clean-eating cookbooks. And that's why she'd reiterated that her family's diet was worlds away from that of her fellow churchgoers. Janae was deeply familiar with the assumptions that I, or any other non-Black researcher, might make about her family. She knew all about the stereotypes associated with them. Janae was adamant that she did not want to be "lumped in," as she put it, with the low-income Black families in my study. "Other people, if they didn't know our color, might think this is a white family," Janae said.

I asked Janae what she meant by that. "Well," she explained, rolling her eyes, "it's a stereotype that all white people are well-off and educated and eating healthy, organic foods and quinoa and all Black people are eating Doritos and getting it from wherever."

I nodded in agreement.

Not all Black people ate those foods, she reminded me. In fact, sometimes white people were the unhealthiest of all. "Go to the state fair," she continued, closing the dishwasher. "We go every year and I've never in my life seen — that's the biggest concentration of low-income white Americans eating fried lard on a stick and diabetic. Like, in the wheelchair eating the lard. Like, 'Your leg is ready to be cut off. And so it's real. Why are you eating fried cheese? And you're white!' And we're Black at the fair eating a cantaloupe stick. But they would never put that. They would put us..."

Janae's voice trailed off, and we stood in silence for a few seconds. I waited for her to finish her sentence, but she never did.

I read Janae's silence, in part, as a sign of her exhaustion. Janae was tired of people making assumptions about what kind of mother she was and what kind of food she fed her kids. She was tired of people concluding, without evidence, that she fed her kids fried chicken and Doritos. And she was tired of having to fend off those and all the other assumptions people made about her as a mom simply because of the color of her skin.

After returning home from Janae's, I flipped open my laptop, opened a new browser window, and navigated to Google Images. I was thinking about the fact that Janae had mentioned multiple times during our conversation how important Michelle Obama's Let's Move! campaign had been for low-income Black communities. I understood her point. The campaign had raised awareness across the country and inspired activism around issues of food justice and childhood obesity. It had also ushered significant resources into Black and brown communities to improve families' nutrition and ease parents' struggles.

But as scholars, advocates, and the media piled onto the movement, a particular imagery had also risen to the surface — an imagery that took on a life of its own and went beyond the original movement's scope or goals. This imagery shaped people's ideas about which children from which communities lacked proper nutrition and which children were obese. That evening, when I typed *Let's Move Childhood Obesity* into my search bar, pictures of Black and Latinx kids flashed across my screen. There were no white kids, only Black and brown. My screen offered proof of what I had suspected: over the years, these kids had become the faces of childhood obesity, the mascots of a public health crisis.

In contrast, to witness our society's glorification of whiteness and thinness, all I needed to do was flip open the latest issue of *Self* magazine in my dentist's office the next week. I looked at the thin, able-bodied blond woman drinking a green smoothie in a remodeled white kitchen, and I juxtaposed this photo with the ones I'd seen earlier of overweight Black children. It made my blood boil to consider how these two starkly different images reinforced a widespread cultural ideology of *healthy* as white and thin and, conversely, *unhealthy* as Black, brown, and overweight.

The day I spent with Janae highlighted just how profoundly racism shapes society's understanding of both healthy eating *and* healthy feeding. Janae was right: When most people thought about childhood obesity, they didn't picture overweight white kids. They envisioned low-income Black kids in a low-income, urban Black neighborhood. This was the stereotype that Janae spent every day of her life pushing back against. It was impossible for me to ignore how fervently, even desperately, she wanted to separate her family from these depictions. Her view of herself as a responsible mother demanded that she distance herself from the pervasive assumptions that she ate unhealthy food and raised unhealthy children.

We live in a country in which people are deemed responsible for their own successes and failures. We applaud parents for their kids' successes and blame them for their kids' failures. When it comes to food, if kids eat well, it's because their moms were active and caring. If kids eat poorly, it's because their moms were lazy and neglectful. The photos of overweight Black and brown kids filling my laptop screen reflected and reinforced untruthful, harmful stereotypes that circulate widely in American society, even if they often go unspoken: that Black and brown moms are bad mothers who don't care about their kids' diets, health, or well-being.

Shutting my laptop, I knew what Janae had been trying to prove to me. I knew how diligently she (and so many other Black and brown parents) had to work to demonstrate that even though she wasn't white, she was still a loving, devoted parent who fed her kids responsibly. That society's depiction of her— and other caregivers of color—wasn't true. That despite the hue of her skin, she was still a good mom.

PART III

Compromises

Rosie was also used to conflicting emotions, for she was a mother and knew every moment of every day that no one out in the world could ever love or value or nurture her children as well as she could and yet that it was necessary nonetheless to send them out into that world anyway.

— LAURIE FRANKEL, *THIS IS HOW IT ALWAYS IS*

CHAPTER 11

Mom's Job

Picture a parent feeding a child. What do you see?

If you're like most people in the United States, the parent you're probably imagining is a mother. Perhaps she is plating her kid's food at a dining-room table. She may be perusing a supermarket with a toddler strapped into the child's seat of a shopping cart. Or maybe she is rifling through the pantry in search of a key dinner ingredient.

If the image of a mother came to mind for you, then your imagination is largely aligned with reality. In the United States, the mom is the parent most likely to be in charge of food. Every day, moms spend, on average, triple the amount of time preparing meals that dads do.[1]

Before beginning this research, I was aware of these national statistics. They made sense to me, aligned as they were with my own personal experiences and observations. I grew up in a family where my mom had been the one to cook meals while my dad had sat down at the table when the meal was ready to be eaten. My dad was handy for a supermarket run and burgers on the grill, but his culinary contributions stopped soon thereafter. I'd seen a similar dynamic play out in friends' and family members' marriages, and I would eventually come to understand its pull within my own marriage and experiences of motherhood. As a woman, I also recognized in myself the myriad ways that I had been socialized to see feeding and nourishing as my responsibility—and even something that made me feel good about myself.

So it was no surprise when I discovered during my research that foodwork in families was gendered and highly unequal. I already knew that moms were overwhelmingly responsible for feeding kids and that dads' involvement was relatively limited.

But the longer I spent at families' sides, the more I realized that an even more important story lay behind the well-known statistics on mothers' and fathers' different time contributions. While these numbers are a key part of what is so unequal, they obscure a key parental dynamic—a dynamic that means moms are often doing even *more* work than national data suggest. Mothers not only spent more time feeding than fathers did; fathers, I found, often increased mothers' feeding-related stresses and frustrations.

Nyah, Dana, Renata, and Julie were like most moms in America: They undertook the work of feeding their kids largely single-handedly. They were the ones in the family who managed the physical and logistical load of keeping everyone nourished. They grocery shopped, restocked fridges and freezers, and threw out expired pantry items. They diced, marinated, sautéed, and baked. They also did feeding's invisible work, from organizing and strategizing to monitoring, worrying, and troubleshooting everyone's diet.

Moms sometimes got help from different family members. I met moms (mostly of color) who harnessed a network of (mostly female) caregivers to help get their kids fed. These were largely mothers who, like 20 percent of the U.S. population, resided in multigenerational homes, as well as moms who lived near extended family.[2] The latter was Dana's situation; Dana's mother, Debra, lived nearby and would sometimes pop over to Dana's place and get dinner started before Dana arrived home from work. I met other moms who enlisted their kids to help with food. Older kids, in particular, were good for boiling pasta, chopping carrots, and swinging by the supermarket to grab a gallon of milk.

But for many moms, the family member closest to them— the husband or the father of their children—offered relatively little help with feeding. Most dads left the lion's share of the daily foodwork to moms.

Of course, this wasn't the case in all of the heterosexual married couples. On one end of the spectrum of paternal involvement was a handful of fathers who were heavily involved in feeding, and some were even the head cooks and primary grocery shoppers in their families. Nationally, about one in ten families have a father who is in charge of both grocery shopping and cooking.[3] Later in the book, I share the experiences of two such dads—Alvaro Morales in chapter 14 and Joaquin Vargas in chapter 17.[4] I also met fathers in the middle of the spectrum who aided moms in making grocery runs, loading the dishwasher, and scrubbing pots and pans. Some of these dads enjoyed cooking but on a recreational basis rather than as routine labor. Brunches and barbecues were where such dads generally took the reins. They could whip up the occasional plate of French toast or host a Sunday grill with a spread of burgers and steaks. On the least-involved end of the spectrum were the dads who were completely uninterested in anything having to do with feeding their families. These dads expressed their dietary preferences to moms, who then had to figure out how to incorporate those preferences with their own and their kids'.[5]

Why were moms generally saddled with most—or all—of the food-related work? One reason is that traditional gender norms dictate that mothers undertake that work. The families I met often had very gendered ideas about moms' instinctual and natural talents for feeding. Many dads told me that moms were inherently better at cooking and all things nutrition-related. They insisted that mothers' "maternal instinct" gave them a natural understanding of what and how their children should be eating. This instinct made mothers better suited to feed kids.[6] As one dad explained, "I'm just a little less... I don't know what the right word is. I don't read about it as much as she might or think about it as much as she might maybe because I'm a guy." Other dads talked about these differences in almost biological terms, as if being a woman was a prerequisite for caring about the food family members ate.

But it wasn't just dads who saw things this way. As we know, foodwork and its relationship to cultivating and protecting children's health are central to motherhood and consistent with intensive mothering's expectation that moms be kids' primary caregivers in all dimensions. Most moms I met didn't question how or why they had fallen into the role of primary food provider, and some described actively seeking it out when they were establishing their families. For moms, being and feeling good required feeding children.

The dads I met, however, didn't need to devote themselves to feeding their kids in order to feel like they were good dads. As core as feeding is to motherhood, it is largely peripheral to fatherhood. While American dads today spend more time with their children than dads did thirty years ago, their involvement in the everyday management of kids' lives and the mundane forms of labor associated with this involvement has continued to lag behind mothers'. Being a good dad in America today has more to do with caretaking activities, like involvement in kids' educational and extracurricular endeavors, than it used to, but what's expected of fathers in terms of food remains extremely limited.[7]

What's more, broad conventional masculinity norms often discourage dads from engaging in healthy behaviors themselves. Research has found that men's lifestyle choices generally include higher rates of risky behaviors that are harmful to health and longevity—for instance, substance abuse and delaying medical care—and lower rates of behaviors that promote optimal health, including dietary behaviors. Indeed, men in the U.S. are less likely to consume a healthy diet than women are. Men's diets are richer in red and processed meats, and men are much less likely than women to be vegetarians. The dads I met told me that their wives generally ate healthier than they did, often offering up gendered explanations for why. As one dad told me, "I am probably less careful than my wife is about what I consume for myself. She's, I think, a little bit more thoughtful and more disciplined about what she'll eat or the portions that she will have. I just thought that, as a guy, maybe I didn't need to pay as much attention." The same norms that guide fathers toward less healthy behaviors can translate into how they care for their children's health. When it comes to food, men's preference for and consumption of a less healthy diet may discourage them from feeling a sense of responsibility for their kids' diets.[8] Indeed, this is what I saw.

One night, Renata and I were prepping dinner in the kitchen before a midweek church service. Renata was making a salad, dicing cucumbers and cherry tomatoes and tossing them into a wide glass bowl of romaine lettuce. I chopped baby carrots into bite-size pieces and added them in handfuls to the mix. Renata grabbed a bottle of Italian vinaigrette from the fridge, poured it over the vegetables, and tossed them delicately with two silver spoons. Then she started working on the garlic bread. She cut the remainder of a baguette into thin slices, then stroked each one with butter and topped it with minced garlic, salt, and dried parsley.

"Does José cook?" I asked her as I put the bag of baby carrots back in the produce drawer. I'd never seen José in the kitchen for longer than the ten seconds it took him to grab a bag of Fritos from the pantry or put a dish in the sink. Renata chuckled and rolled her eyes as she slid the bread into the preheated oven.

José knew how to cook a few things, she said, but he preferred her to cook because she knew more recipes.

"He can put a pot of rice on the stove," she told me, putting a few dirty dishes into the sink to soak. "If I call him on my way home and tell him to put a pot of rice on, he can do that."

Most often, Renata prepared José's food. Another evening, before José left to perform a show with his band, Renata had made him two roast beef and cheese sandwiches on white bread and zipped them up in a lunch box along with a bag of chips. It was how she prepared the kids' lunches too, and it made me wonder if Renata ever felt like she had three kids to feed rather than two. Tonight, she said, sighing with relief, José would either grab fast food before church or eat leftovers after the service.

While we were on the topic of men and cooking, Renata mentioned a friend whose boyfriend loved to cook. "She's so lucky!" Renata laughed, turning the oven light on and kneeling down to check on the garlic bread. If Renata wasn't home, José would pick up the kids, Renata said, and then go to the drive-through because "it's quick and it's easy to do. He thinks that he did what he needed to do." I could see why: José's goal was getting the kids fed, and the drive-through was an obvious way to check that box. But buying the kids fast food was not what Renata thought he should do. For Renata, the drive-through was a cop-out. It was a last resort, not a first choice. Renata thought that when she wasn't home, José should make sure the kids ate some vegetables. He needed to reflect on what he was teaching them every time he let them eat junk. José, Renata thought, needed to stop making her life harder.

To be clear, José and other dads were not deliberately trying to frustrate moms or compromise their children's diets. The dads I met were loving, committed caregivers who wanted the best for their children. Nonetheless, dads largely felt absolved of responsibility for their children's diets.[9] This absolution could lead dads to inadvertently undermine moms' efforts. Dads were more likely to relax boundaries or ignore rules moms struggled to uphold. Dads were more inclined to take kids to the drive-through and say yes to chips and soda. Dads took a more laid-back approach to food and were willing to go with the flow when moms would have preferred them to lay down the law.

What was striking to me about fathers' undermining attitudes and behaviors was that they rarely seemed malicious, or even intentional. It was almost like dads were clueless about how much additional stress they inflicted on moms when they undercut moms' efforts. In fact, many dads seemed completely unaware of how deeply and emotionally invested moms were in their kids' diets.

But this was exactly the issue. The problem for moms wasn't just that dads did less of the foodwork; by caring less about their kids' intake, dads also amplified moms' anxieties and added to moms' labor. José's behavior and Renata's reaction were common among the families I met. Other dads mirrored José in their willingness to feed kids less healthy food. Other moms noticed, as Renata did, their husbands' tendencies, which then became an additional source of stress. Dads added even more balls to moms' already untenable juggling act. In addition to having to navigate and negotiate kids' unhealthy preferences, moms had to worry about whether dads were further derailing kids' diets—and then figure out if and when to intervene.

When dads treated kids to fast food or indulged their requests for candy, moms felt that their hard work was being undone. Watching dads say yes to the very things they were working so hard to say no to felt like a punch in the gut to moms. It made them feel that, even in a pinch, they could not rely on fathers to feed kids with the required amount of care and intentionality. They couldn't depend on dads to track or intervene in kids' diets as necessary. They couldn't even trust dads to put together healthy lunches for kids if moms were otherwise occupied. Moms knew this simple, frustrating truth: if they didn't monitor what their kids ate, no one would.

This feeling mothers had of exclusive responsibility—of always being on the hook, even if they weren't physically there—upped the already high stakes for them. There was no respite from feeding, and there was rarely a day off. Moms had to keep track of what went into and came out of the fridge, monitoring stock and making shopping lists. Each mom was the family grocer, restocker, shopper, head chef, line cook, and server. She had to figure out how to vary lunch-box contents and plan out dinners. When the egg carton was empty, she had to go to the supermarket or remind someone else to swing by. When kids left for school without eating breakfast, Mom was the one running behind with a granola bar or piece of fruit. When someone refused to eat peas, Mom did the negotiating at the dinner table.

Many moms complained about fathers when it came to food. Julie, for instance, was annoyed that Zach was rarely home for dinner and that he would stock up on items from Costco that ended up going to waste because he chose the wrong things. It wasn't the cost that bothered her; it was Zach's lack of concern for what their family actually liked to eat.

"He'll buy stuff from Costco that he knows I'll never use," Julie said, rolling her eyes. "It goes bad, it gets freezer burn, and I throw it in the trash." One Wednesday before heading out for a long girls' weekend, Julie walked me through the plan she'd worked out for family meals in her absence. "Zach will probably take the kids out for dinner on Thursday and Friday because he does not know how to cook." Julie looked down at the calendar on her phone as she scrolled through the days she'd be gone. "They'll make their lunches. And then I have a friend coming to watch them on Saturday and Sunday. I'll have stuff for her to make—chicken or pasta, the standard go-to." Julie paused. "The kids will eat. They just might not eat a vegetable at every meal."

Zach agreed with Julie's take. He once told me that he didn't really get involved with Evan's or Jane's diet. It was Julie's job, and Zach just pinch-hit when absolutely necessary. "I only pay attention to what the kids eat when I'm here or when we're all out traveling," he said.

Zach also figured that when he *had* to feed the kids—if Julie wasn't around for some reason—he didn't have to think too much about what they ate. Because moms were so diligent most of the time about setting and enforcing the rules, it wasn't a big deal if dads broke them once in a while. What this meant for moms was that dads were essentially always off the hook.

Stay-at-home moms saw dads' laissez-faire approaches to feeding differently than working moms did. While Julie found Zach's lack of interest in food, cooking, and shared meals annoying, she felt largely resigned to that reality. Because of the clear division of labor that came with being the stay-at-home parent, Julie saw feeding as a central part of her job. It would have been nice if Zach contributed or took more of an interest in food, but Julie never expected it. She was okay with this responsibility resting on her shoulders and with Zach being a player in his kids' diets only when it was convenient for him.

Compared to Julie, working mothers like Renata were often visibly more frustrated by the unequal division of labor. Even in families where both parents were employed full-time, moms still took on most of the feeding.[10] Renata felt that José did little, if anything, to help when it came to feeding the family. That responsibility rested squarely on Renata's shoulders, something that had to be done in addition to working full-time and shuttling the kids around—commitments that kept Renata out of the house from at least seven a.m. to six p.m. most weekdays and many weekends as well.

One thing I admired about Renata was her understated optimism. Renata was genuinely thankful for everything God

had given her. Even when she described life's hurdles and incon-
veniences, she did so almost matter-of-factly; complaining or
whining wasn't her style. Because of Renata's usually positive
disposition, I noticed on the evening that we prepared a salad
and garlic bread that she seemed unusually, visibly irritated.

Renata was frustrated with José's giving the kids fast food
because she knew there was no real solution. As far as feeding the
kids was concerned, her and José's arrangement was likely not a
negotiable one. So instead of trying to change things, Renata
worked to make light of the situation. "It's a joke to us, like, 'No
more fatty patties.'" She imitated herself scolding José, forcing a
laugh. "'Quit going through the McDonald's drive-through!'"

But Renata was actually more irritated than tickled. If José
was going to be swaying the kids' diets in a negative direction, it
meant Renata *really* had to feed them well the rest of the time.
Doing all the grocery shopping and cooking was hard enough.
But on top of this, if she wanted to establish healthy habits for
her kids, she had to go the extra mile to offset José's unhealthy
dietary influence.

Still, like other moms, Renata sometimes reluctantly took
cues from José, allowing his less healthy preferences and his
penchant for fast food to win out. Just as it could be easier to say
yes to her kids' food requests than to fight a battle, following
José's lead offered the path of least resistance. A few weeks back,
Renata had returned home after a long day at work, dropped
her purse by the front door, and collapsed onto the living-room
sofa. Although bone-tired, she was still planning to cook dinner.
The pasta ingredients were waiting in the fridge. But then José
offered her an alternative. "Do you just wanna go get pizza?" he
asked hopefully.

Renata usually disliked José's eagerness to order takeout.
But that night, she mostly felt a sense of relief about not having
to make dinner for everyone. They ordered two pizzas, and
Renata ate cross-legged on the couch with the TV on. It was

luxurious. But later, Renata felt guilty about letting José steer her family toward a less nutritious dinner.

Renata paused after telling me this story. Then she pulled the garlic bread out of the oven and said, "We really gotta limit our fast-food intake."

Try as Renata might not to worry so much about what her family ate, she couldn't tamp down the stress that arose when she fell short of feeding them healthy, homemade meals. Maybe José didn't need to nourish the kids to feel like a good parent, but as a mom, Renata didn't have that luxury. When she gave in to either her kids' or José's requests, she struggled with the maternal guilt that quickly ensued. Even in her most exhausted state, even when there wasn't time to cook, and even when Renata told herself it shouldn't be her responsibility alone, in her mind, the facts remained the same — it *was* Renata's responsibility to keep the family nourished. And if she didn't do it, no one else would. The next evening, Renata made sure to prepare a homemade meal of chicken, pasta, and salad.

CHAPTER 12

Time and Money

"I've always worked," Delfina Carrillo, the single mom of fifteen-year-old Luis, told me. Her full-time job as a supermarket cashier, Delfina explained, was one key reason why Luis's diet diverged so sharply from hers growing up.

"My mom never worked." Delfina sighed, pushing her wire-framed glasses back on her nose. Delfina's mom, who had raised Delfina and her siblings, had spent hours in the kitchen each day rolling yellow and blue corn tortillas and making pots of *posole* and *caldo de pollo*. Delfina, however, had worked as a cashier for twenty-six years, laboring for ten hours a day on her feet. By the time her shift wrapped up, at half past six in the evening, cooking a homemade meal was the absolute last thing Delfina wanted to do. She was mentally and physically beat, with aching soles from standing and a gnawing headache from fending off customer complaints from dawn till dusk.[1]

"I'd call the kids up after work and say, 'You know what?'" Delfina took a sip of water. "'I'm tired. What do you want? I'll pick it up.'" Other nights, Delfina would just grab a pepperoni pizza from the freezer aisle before driving home. Pizza was always a safe bet.

Talking with Delfina about work underscored just how physically distinct low-income moms' jobs were from wealthier moms'—and how much that affected their food choices. Delfina's job was extremely physically taxing. I met other moms who worked as cashiers, clerks, childcare providers, home-health aides, house cleaners, dishwashers, restaurant servers, baristas, or line cooks, and many of them spent eight to twelve hours a day standing, walking, pushing, pulling, and carrying. Compared to the careers of many wealthier working mothers, these moms' jobs taxed their bodies for hours without rest and with minimal breaks.

For Delfina, coming home to toil over a hot stove or hunch over a cutting board demanded even more physical exertion. It sometimes felt like too much—like the straw that might finally, actually break her back. When Delfina was married, she worked fewer hours and had more energy at the end of the day. She would generally cook at least a few evenings a week. But when her husband left, she started putting in longer hours to make ends meet. She went from working forty hours a week to sixty. She dragged herself home most evenings feeling more depleted than ever.

"It's hard to explain." Delfina exhaled. "But I didn't want to spend all my time just cooking and cooking and cleaning and doing, doing, doing. I kind of wanted to spend some time with Luis and then have some downtime for myself too, you know?"

Delfina's desire to spend time with her child and have a moment for herself was widely shared by moms across income levels. But low-income moms, who endured longer, less flexible, and more physically demanding work shifts than moms with high-income jobs, found it hard to achieve this balance while pulling together the homemade meals they felt they should be cooking. They were well aware that good moms cooked dinner. But many also felt, like Delfina, that good moms spent quality time with their kids. So on weekday evenings, when Delfina walked back through the front door and knew that she had just a couple of hours to catch up with her son, there was a hard decision to be made. Did she spend those precious moments standing in the kitchen chopping bell peppers and peeling potatoes, or did she sidle up on the sofa beside Luis to catch a few moments in his company?

When it comes to public discussions of healthy eating, time is a well-known issue. It's common knowledge that a lack of time is a major barrier to eating nutritiously. When time is short, cooking is one of the first things to go out the window. The hours that it takes to visit the supermarket, prep ingredients, cook a meal, and wash pots and pans are ones that many of us don't have. And because of that time scarcity, we turn to quicker, more convenient, and less healthy options, and our diets can suffer.

For families especially, time has become tighter than ever. For one thing, parents work longer hours and commute longer distances than they used to. For another, today there are more mothers in the workforce and more mothers raising children as single parents than there used to be.[2] These two trends mean that many families today no longer have a parent with ample time to devote to feeding. Even though, as I highlighted in the prior chapter, moms were still generally the ones getting everyone fed, most moms didn't have much time to devote to the cause. Rather, they fit shopping and cooking into their busy working and caregiving schedules where they could.

Just as pervasive as discussions about time scarcity are supposed antidotes to it. The internet is full of solutions or life hacks that highlight ways to cut corners or plan ahead so you can still pull off homemade healthy meals, even in a time crunch. Magazines feature articles with headlines like "Twelve Ways to Eat Healthy No Matter How Busy You Are" and "How to Eat Healthy When You Don't Have Time to Meal Prep." The market is flooded with cookbooks with titles like *Weeknight Wonders: Delicious, Healthy Dinners in Thirty Minutes or Less* and *The Quick and Easy Healthy Cookbook.* Moms are a special target of this messaging, with parenting blogs featuring posts like "Seventy-Two Easy Kid-Friendly Dinners Perfect for Weeknights" and "A

Week of Healthy Kids Meal Ideas (That Actually Work in Real Life)."[3]

The take-home message is clear: If you have a half hour, then a healthy, homemade meal is possible. Of course, the pre- and post-work of cooking and the time required to grocery shop and clean up are rarely included in this half hour. But more important, these relatively simplistic discussions of time generally ignore one of its essential components: quality.

Certainly, time is a quantifiable resource, measured in seconds, minutes, hours, and days. But time also has a rich qualitative element to it—time can be enjoyable, stressful, restorative, or exhausting. You evaluate how well spent your time is based on these kinds of qualities. When you reflect on how you currently spend your days and consider how to spend them moving forward, you may ask yourself: What is the best use of my time?

This question bears directly on food choices, and yet it's one that is rarely, if ever, discussed with any nuance. Cooking a healthy meal, according to the prevailing wisdom, is time well spent. But the reality for moms, I learned, wasn't so clear-cut.

For moms who were pressed for time, cooking meals came with real, tangible trade-offs—especially when those meals were supposed to come together quickly on a weeknight after a long day of work and school. Those trade-offs had everything to do with the quality of the time these moms got to spend with their children.

In general, moms' decision to cook *more* entailed a choice to spend *less* recreational time with kids and on themselves. It meant feeling *more* exhausted than they already felt and even *less* connected to the kids whom they hadn't seen all day.

Delfina explained that when she let Luis eat what he liked, she enjoyed their time together more. Her son was fed and happy, and the two had longer to hang out. What's more, that time together was way more pleasant. Occasionally, Delfina devoted the time she saved by not cooking to helping Luis with his homework. Often, the two kicked back and watched a sitcom together. But whatever the case, for Delfina, the quality of that time together surpassed that of laboring over a frying pan.

Driving home from Delfina's, I kept thinking about how time wasn't a resource that only low-income moms lacked—moms across the income spectrum were generally busy and harried. All working moms were overbooked, whether they were cashiers like Delfina or had jobs as dentists, teachers, or lawyers. Some held down multiple jobs, and many were gone more than forty hours a week. But stay-at-home moms like Julie were also really busy. Julie often had difficulty finding time to schedule me in amid all her household responsibilities, volunteering activities, social engagements, and shuttling. One week, she texted that she couldn't find a single time for me to stop by.

But there was one important difference. Compared to working moms who struggled to find time to shop, cook, and clean up, Julie embraced food as a critical use of her time. Because Julie had spent the past seventeen years as her children's full-time caregiver, food was neither an afterthought nor something to squeeze in on the evenings and weekends—it was her daily work. It was a key part of her job, and she tackled it with professional ambition. Whether it was making multiple trips to the supermarket in a day or preparing dinners specifically requested by Evan and Jane, Julie devoted herself to the cause of her children's diets. And when she saw her home-cooked meals grace her kids' plates, she felt fulfilled. When Julie watched Jane eat one rather than four cookies or Evan order a salad, Julie found proof that the hours she devoted to feeding her kids each week was time—and energy—well spent.

I witnessed firsthand Julie's temporal investment in food. One week, she drove to the supermarket four times to make sure that the fridge was stocked with Jane's favorite healthy snack: red and green grapes. Julie's time is what allowed her to make sure that Jane always had fresh fruit to eat and not just bags of chips. Another evening, I spent hours helping Julie prepare a side dish especially for Jane: a "tornado potato" dish made from spiral slicing, skewering, and roasting potatoes in a homemade sauce. Sometimes, Julie was exhausted by her efforts and even found the task a little thankless. But she also saw it as her job, and Julie took her job seriously.

But not all high-income moms had as much time as Julie to devote to food. *How are these moms making it work?* I wondered. What I learned was that in the absence of time, money could mean the difference between a more or less nutritious meal.

"It's more stressful than I would like," Sonali Kapoor, a mom of two, told me about feeding her family of four. I met Sonali and her husband, Arjun, one evening in their spacious two-story house at the end of a quiet cul-de-sac. Their street was lined with other two-million-dollar homes, each with a white façade, a brown thatched roof, and a neatly manicured front lawn. Arjun, a short man with thick black hair and a well-trimmed mustache, opened the door.

"Come on in," he said. I removed my shoes in the entryway and followed him into a bright living area with high ceilings and broad windows that faced the backyard. An open-concept kitchen flowed into a beige and white den. Sonali, her thick brown hair swept into a neat bun, stood by the kitchen sink, rinsing plates from dinner and loading them into the dishwasher. The Kapoor boys—sixteen-year-old Zubin and nine-year-old Dev—had already retreated upstairs to get ready for bed.

The first thing I noticed about Arjun and Sonali, still both in their gray and black business-casual attire, was that behind their upbeat exteriors lay exhaustion. I could almost feel the heaviness of Sonali's eyelids as she took a seat by their fireplace and pulled a thick blanket over her legs. Arjun sank into the chair next to her. I sat across from them on a tan sofa, my cup of water on the glass coffee table.

Sonali and Arjun had grown up in India, where they'd met as graduate students. They married and then moved to North America—first to Canada and later to the Bay Area. "Education was very, very important and so we got educated," Arjun explained. Once they had their degrees in hand, their careers had taken off—Sonali now ran the marketing department of a large tech company, and Arjun was in charge of a global firm's human resources office.

The Kapoors' diet, however, felt far less successful to Sonali. When the Kapoors first arrived in the United States, American food culture was a shock to their systems. Growing up in India, Sonali and Arjun ate nothing but fresh food. Both of their mothers, stay-at-home caregivers, bought fruits and vegetables daily from the market and prepared three meals a day using fresh produce. Sonali and Arjun had both been raised in vegetarian households, where okra, paneer, and lentils were staples.

Sonali and Arjun felt that their current lives were a far cry from that. "I think the biggest differences from back then," Arjun said, "are that we don't eat as much fresh food so there's a lot of processed food or leftovers. And we tend to eat out I'd say about thirty percent of the time or so."

These differences weighed on Sonali and irked her more than they did Arjun. "Too often, convenience kicks in for us," Sonali lamented, bringing a glass of water to her lips. Daily supermarket trips and nightly meals from scratch were out of the question. For Sonali, it all came down to time. She simply didn't have enough of it. Both she and Arjun commuted to work, and the boys were enrolled at two different schools. Between drop-offs, pickups, Bay Area traffic, and extracurriculars, the Kapoors were constantly on the go. While moms like Julie had mornings and afternoons to shop and prepare family meals,

Sonali had only the weekends. But spending all her time shopping and cooking on Saturday and Sunday came at a cost. Those were the only two days the family could spend quality time together.

"I have to choose between being together and making food," Sonali said, sighing.

On Saturdays, Zubin and Dev attended Hindu school. The school was about a forty-five-minute drive from their home. Arjun could easily take them, and Sonali could use the time to shop and meal prep for the week. But splitting up had its downsides. The boys would be gone for four to five hours while Sonali worked alone in the kitchen. Since Sonali barely caught glimpses of her husband and children during the week, she decided to forgo weekend meal-prep time and instead ride along to Hindu school so that the four of them could spend time in one another's company. "Even if we are in the car," Sonali said, smiling, "at least we are together."

Many lower-income families were also short on time, but the Kapoors had a key extra resource: money. Families like Sonali and Arjun's could throw cash at the problem of time scarcity. Everything, from shopping to prepping to cooking, could be outsourced. The outsourcing strategy I saw families use most frequently was grocery delivery. But I also met those who relied on meal companies that delivered premeasured raw ingredients that could be transformed into a dinner in fifteen minutes. Other families used services that delivered the meals already cooked and ready to be reheated. And some families even hired personal chefs or a "mother's helper" to prepare meals in their kitchens. The Kapoors decided to give this last option a try.

"The solution," Sonali told me, "is that somebody comes on Sunday morning to make food." That somebody's name was Dipika, and she had years of experience preparing North Indian cuisine. Paying Dipika to cook left Sonali with just enough control—Sonali still did the grocery shopping and picked the recipes, but Dipika minced garlic, ginger, and onions and kneaded dough. Dipika was essentially Sonali's sous-chef. Because Dipika stood over a warm stove for hours while the spices and bases for dishes simmered, Sonali could devote her time to other things.

When I spoke with the Kapoors a few months into this new arrangement, they told me that it was working well for them. It freed Sonali on the weekends to spend more hours with her sons. While Sonali didn't love how Dipika prepared some of the dishes, the outsourcing allowed her to check a bunch of boxes that mattered to her. Healthy, Indian, home-cooked meals: check. Time to spend with the rest of the family: check.[4]

The Kapoors weren't the only ones with this idea. Sonali explained that Dipika worked for a handful of other South Asian families in the area. After spending the early hours of Sunday morning in the Kapoors' kitchen, Dipika would travel to four or five other homes throughout the day to help other moms get a head start on the week. Sometimes Dipika brought her own assistant, which allowed her to work with even greater speed and pay more families a visit in one day.

Outsourcing also gave wealthier moms more bandwidth to say no to their kids' food requests when they had to. It gave them that extra bit of patience to refuse when their kids asked for Pepsi or Snickers. In this way, having money helped not just because it enabled parents to buy more expensive food and save time while not sacrificing quality; it also gave parents the internal strength to wage yearslong battles to keep their kids' diets as nutritious as possible. Before her helper had come on board, Sonali had often been so tired at the end of the day that the last thing she wanted to do was argue with Dev about whether he could have ice cream for dessert. Her situation has echoed Delfina's in this way. But with a little time and a bit of energy freed up, Sonali could more often summon the will to negotiate. Her resources gave her that extra buffer to keep going—to keep striving to improve her sons' diets. Sonali didn't regret paying someone else to cook instead of cooking herself. That investment was what kept her and her family on track.

When I compared Delfina's situation to Sonali's, I saw how resources like time and money could come together to make it easier for some families to eat healthier than others. Having both resources gave more privileged families an obvious advantage. But in a pinch, one resource in particular could compensate for the other—money remained the key currency for opening doors. Money solved problems, allowing mothers to creatively devise strategies to overcome obstacles to healthy eating. Money let moms order in, take out, hire help, and do more with fewer hours in the day. Money, quite literally, bought moms quality time to spend with their children. It bought them more bandwidth and energy to keep working at their children's diets. It bought them healthier food without *all* the effort. When time was lacking, I learned, money could always compensate.

CHAPTER 13

Stuck

Renata didn't have the money to compensate for time scarcity. Her situation diverged from that of more affluent moms. To the outside world, the difference between a mom like Renata and a mom like Julie wasn't always obvious. Both were married. Both were devoted mothers to a son and daughter. Both were raising kids who were happy, busy, and excelling in school. There was no question that Renata and her family lived relatively comfortably. Like Julie, Renata was able to get her kids many things that they wanted, whether it was new back-to-school clothes or the dog they'd been asking for for months. And when it came to food, both Julie and Renata thought and cared about what their kids ate. They wanted their kids to be healthy, and they used the resources they had at their disposal to help make that happen.

But I was also struck by the visible distinctions between the approaches each took to feed her family. Compared to Julie, Renata was always being forced to make compromises. Not the kind of daily compromises that Nyah and Dana had to make, but compromises that left Renata feeling inadequate — especially when she juxtaposed them with her vision of a good mom. As was the case for other middle-class moms, the trade-offs demanded by Renata's situation left her feeling stuck. With more limited time and money, she couldn't figure out how exactly to feed her kids the way she aspired to.

Some of Renata's compromises stemmed from her full-time

job and evenings spent shuttling the kids to their various activities. All of this exhausted and fragmented Renata, often leaving her too depleted to feel excited about whipping up a gourmet dinner. In this way, her lifestyle paralleled Sonali's, whose demanding job also rendered her less bandwidth to devote to food.

But Sonali's and Renata's situations diverged from there. Sonali had the money to outsource some of her load, thereby wrangling back some of that bandwidth. Renata, however, didn't have the money to outsource the cognitive or physical load of cooking. Renata somehow, and often largely on her own, had to make it work.

"Our busy schedules sort of guide how we eat," Renata explained to me one morning. Because of that, Renata tended to prepare the same simple meals over and over again, ones she knew by heart and that she could get on the dinner table in less than fifteen minutes. She wasn't spending hours perusing recipes online, delving into cookbooks to try out new meals, or watching cooking tutorials on Instagram. Renata was all about familiar, fail-safe recipes that could be popped in the microwave or oven at the last minute. She was about efficiency. On the nights she was totally exhausted, Renata opted for pizza delivery.

Sometimes, I felt like I could almost *see* the gap between Renata's dietary aspirations and her reality. The Ortegas' fridge was often filled with stacks of takeout boxes and restaurant doggie bags. One Tuesday evening, I spotted two Papa John's pizza boxes and some Panda Express containers peeking out of the recycling bin. Renata, I knew, was one of the modern mothers whom the food industry had in mind when it came up with processed products—the supposed "solutions" to moms' desire to feed their kids nutritiously, quickly, and without complaints. But these solutions generally only left Renata feeling guilty about the shortcuts she'd had to take to get there.

Renata's guilt was usually highest when it came to giving the kids processed foods. One afternoon, as Renata and I drove Amalia to the pediatrician, we talked about Amalia's love of mac and cheese. "It's our favorite," Amalia chimed in from the back seat over the sound of pop music on the radio.

"And I feel bad giving it to them," Renata quickly added as we turned into the parking lot. Renata found processed products overly artificial, with the powdery cheese and expiration date years out. At the same time, Renata didn't want to just outright refuse the kids' requests. After all, it was an easy dinner to put together and a surefire crowd-pleaser. It was also a simple way for Renata to show them she was listening to their preferences. Renata's compromise? Stove-top mac and cheese, rather than the microwaveable version. It had more real cheese and less of the artificial stuff.

Were these meals exciting? Renata didn't think so. Were they *exactly* what she wanted her kids to be eating? Not quite. But were they nutritious enough? Could they be put together in the time she had? Did they get the job done? The answers were yes, yes, and yes. For Renata, that had to do.

Feeling stuck complicated food's meaning to Renata and other middle-class moms. These moms were precariously trapped between competing ideals and pressures around what it meant to be a good mom. Renata aspired to have as many home-cooked meals as Julie and as many "teaching moments" as Patricia Adams, but having fewer resources barred her from that reality.

As I spent time with wealthier moms who had so much of what Renata wanted, I began to imagine how more resources could change how Renata felt about feeding. This was on my mind one Wednesday evening in August when I met Renata at home. Outside, it felt like summer; at half past six, the air was warm and the sun shone high in the sky. But inside, summer was officially over—almost. Tomorrow was the kids' first day back at school. Amalia would be starting tenth grade and Nico eighth.

Amalia sat at the dining-room table in jean shorts and a blue tank top, tapping away on her iPhone screen.

Renata was sorting the family's mail into two piles, one to keep and one to toss. "The plan tonight is to go to the mall," Renata told me, occasionally glancing up from the pile of papers. Placing her hand on Amalia's shoulder, she smiled. "Amalia needs some new clothes for school." Amalia grinned without looking up from her phone.

Grabbing the pile of mail to toss with her left hand, Renata motioned to me with her right to follow her into the kitchen. The Ortegas' kitchen was narrow and densely packed. On the four-burner stove sat a colander and a small saucepan. Renata picked the colander up and scraped a knotted clump of day-old angel-hair pasta into the trash. Then she grabbed the handle of the saucepan, brought it over to the sink, and filled it with warm water. She used a sponge to wash the tomato residue out, then placed the wet pan upside down on the countertop to dry.

On the top of the fridge was a double box of Honey Bunches of Oats and a six-pack of pale ale. Between the microwave and fridge, a half-eaten loaf of wheat bread was covered in plastic.

"Nico is going to start making his sandwiches for school this year," Renata said, noticing me eyeing the bread. She seemed relieved. "I just want both kids to be in charge of their lunches so I don't have to worry about it."

Rolling up my sleeves, I asked what was for dinner that night and how I could help.

"Amalia isn't hungry," Renata told me, adding that her daughter had biked that afternoon to the local pizza place. "But we can make something for Nico now, and then Amalia can eat some of it later if she wants."

Renata opened the fridge and scanned the shelves to see what she had. Then she reached into the freezer, grabbed two pork cutlets wrapped in plastic, and started defrosting them in the microwave. Amid the hum of the microwave, the two of us talked about how hard it was to line up everyone's schedules so that they could share a meal in the evenings. The kids each had different extracurricular activities, and in his off-hours, José played with the band. Sometimes he was home in the evenings, but that wasn't something Renata could count on.

"It's okay that we don't eat together," she assured me. "I have enough to worry about, I don't need to be getting everyone on different schedules all synced up." I couldn't tell if Renata actually believed that or if she was trying to convince herself—or me. She didn't need to convince me. From where I was sitting, Renata's approach made perfect sense for her family. Everyone was busy, and I had witnessed how frustrating it was for moms to spend so many hours cooking only to find out that one kid had already eaten with friends or another had stopped liking a certain food. Renata was, above all, pragmatic.

But pragmatism wasn't a tenet of intensive mothering, and Renata often felt like she wasn't doing enough. She walked to the end of their long galley kitchen and opened a door to reveal a narrow pantry lined with crackers, fruit cups, canned tomatoes, chips, cereal boxes, and soda. She picked up a large bag of long-grain white rice, carried it back to the counter, plopped it down, and opened it up. She combined two cups of dry rice with four cups of water in a saucepan and set it to cook.

As Renata pulled the defrosted pork cutlets out of the microwave and started to sear them in a nonstick frying pan, she told me about a fantasy she had been entertaining. That fantasy, it turned out, was Sonali's reality. It was a fantasy about getting unstuck.

Renata prefaced it with "I know it's not realistic." She pursed her lips. "But my dream would be to hire someone who could get home a bit before me, start tidying up, and cook us dinner." That person, Renata explained, would change everything for her. It's not that Renata minded grocery shopping or popping something in the oven. And sure, in a world where she had afternoons to chop and prep, she could imagine spending an hour getting things ready for the evening. But that wasn't Renata's reality. Instead, she generally came home after a long and stressful day to a messy kitchen and had to do what she was doing tonight: cleaning up, defrosting, cooking something new, serving everyone, and cleaning up again.

Looking longingly down at the pan, Renata flipped over a pork cutlet.

"That would be the best." She sighed, smiling to herself. Then she started telling me about a friend who had recently hired a caretaker for her kids. But, Renata added excitedly, that caretaker went above and beyond, cleaning the house and cooking full meals for the family. She could make lasagnas, tacos, and even gourmet salads.

"Now, that's what I want!" Renata proclaimed, passing me a cucumber to chop. I peeled, seeded, and sliced the cucumber, wondering if Renata could or would actually hire someone to make her life easier.

"Do you think you could do something like that?" I asked, scraping the cucumber slices from the cutting board into a bowl.

Renata paused, setting the spatula down on the counter for a second. "You know, it's not really in our budget," she said, her disappointment lingering in the air. The Ortegas had just bought a puppy, and both kids were hoping to go on a school trip to Washington, DC, that summer. "But I don't know," she continued. "Maybe it could actually be worth it."

Renata was quiet for a few minutes as she poured two tablespoons of soy sauce into the pan. The black liquid popped and sizzled as it flavored the cutlets. Turning the stove off, she seemed to be actively calculating whether she and José could swing it.

I did my own math. Assuming someone like that cost around thirty dollars an hour and would be needed two hours a day, five days a week, that added up to about twelve hundred dollars a month. If they used the money they would receive as compensation for participating in my research—which was three hundred dollars—they could afford a helper for…one week.

While it would make a world of difference in Renata's life, I couldn't see them putting down over fourteen grand a year to make it happen. I couldn't even imagine them paying half that amount. Renata knew that too—which was why she felt stuck. She definitely didn't love cooking and she didn't *want* to be spending her time on food. She had so many other interests she'd rather have pursued with any extra time, whether it was practicing a dance routine with Amalia or lying on the couch watching the Olympics women's swimming finals. But Renata also felt like she needed to be making at least a few homemade meals each week for her kids. She couldn't subvert that feeling enough to abandon the whole endeavor. She couldn't overcome the guilt.

"I do it," Renata explained about cooking, "because I have to." Renata felt trapped between how she *wanted* to feel about feeding her family and how she *actually* felt about it. Good moms loved cooking and nourishing their families. Good moms never resented chopping cucumbers or deboning a chicken. Cooking should have been a source of joy or satisfaction in her life, Renata thought. But it just wasn't. More than that, it was stressful constantly looking for things to feed her kids that they liked, were nutritious, and wouldn't keep her in the kitchen for hours. Renata told me that some of her friends, also moms, cooked nightly for their families. "They find it therapeutic," she said, flashing me a look of incredulity. "They love to try new recipes, and they love to have lots of friends over to eat their food." Renata paused. "I am *not* one of those people."

After scooping the pork cutlets onto a plate, Renata checked to see if the rice was ready. "This will get us through tonight and tomorrow," she said with relief. As she started to clean up, Renata shouted to Nico that his dinner was ready. Nico sauntered into the kitchen in a black T-shirt and blue jeans, a pair of headphones around his neck. Renata heaped two spoonfuls of white rice, a pork cutlet, and a large helping of cucumbers onto his plate. As she did that, Nico reached into the fridge, grabbed a gallon carton of milk from the lower shelf, and poured himself a tall glass. He took both the plate and the glass into the dining room to eat.

For a moment, Renata felt good. She leaned back onto the counter with a sense of accomplishment. In just under an hour, she had done what she needed to do to get the kids fed and have leftovers for the next few days. Paired with other foods Renata had on hand, the pork, rice, and cucumbers would last through Friday, easily. But as she started to scrub the dirty pan in the sink, she glanced at the microwave clock. "Oh, shoot!" she said, turning the faucet off. "Nico," she called, "I have to rush you because the mall is closing soon, and we have to go." Nico had barely taken his first bite, but he shoveled a few scoops of rice and meat into his mouth before picking his plate back up and walking it into the kitchen.

Grabbing her purse off the table, Renata ushered us out. The mall was closing in less than an hour, but we managed to stop by Forever 21 and Hollister and pick up a pair of shorts and two shirts for Amalia. By the time we got home, it was nine o'clock and Renata was completely wiped. While Amalia showed off her clothes to her dad at the dining-room table, Renata collapsed onto the large beige sofa in the den. Crossing one leg over the other and letting her eyes close for a second, she sighed. "I'll clean the kitchen up tomorrow."

Later that night, back home scarfing down a late dinner at my own kitchen island, I typed up my field notes from the evening.

"Renata is keeping her head above water, but she's also making so many compromises," I wrote. It was true; she was giving her all to everyone. She juggled work, family, and everything that so predictably fell on moms when it came to food. But without extra resources to make that juggling act a little easier, middle-income moms like Renata were all on their own to pull it off. Renata was forced to make trade-offs that left her feeling a sense of guilt and inadequacy. And, as I'd soon learn, she was in good company.

CHAPTER 14

Fluctuating Finances

As a society, our image of middle-class families is that they are, for the most part, financially stable and secure. This image reflects nostalgia more than reality, as the stability that used to characterize the American middle class has been dwindling over the past forty years. The term *middle class* used to refer to Americans who had a steady income, a home, and savings for the future. But today, as the journalist Anne Helen Petersen has pointed out, being middle class mostly means being able to put bills on autopay and service one's debt. Middle-class wages have increased over time, but those increases mostly keep pace with inflation rather than with the rising costs of living in the U.S. More of middle-class paychecks now goes to covering basic expenses, like out-of-pocket health-care fees, childcare, and educational investments.[1]

While the American middle class continues to buy and lease cars, purchase homes (though not at the rate they used to), go on vacation, and pay for kids' education and activities, they are now doing so by taking on significant debt. Indeed, rates of middle-class debt have soared. In March 2020, household debt in the U.S. was $14.3 trillion and student-loan debt was $1.56 trillion, with the average student-debt load for an individual just above $32,000.

Many of the middle-class families I met reflected this reality. While their education placed them culturally in the middle class, their wages and accumulated debt could locate them just above the poverty line. This meant they were both scraping by *and* earning too much to qualify for government aid. For some, attending college had been a double-edged sword; on the one hand, it had propelled them into higher-paying jobs. But on the other, it had saddled them with payments they never seemed to be able to get fully on top of.

Of all the middle-class families I met, Renata and José seemed to be doing the best. They didn't feel financially secure, but they were faring relatively well. They were contributing toward retirement savings. They had health insurance. They owned their three-bedroom house and were regularly making their mortgage payments. They weren't paying off student loans. They could also afford to cover an emergency expense. But other middle-income families were not as lucky, and for those families, unexpected job losses or medical fees laid bare their hidden financial insecurities.

Middle-class families could find their financial situations fluctuating dramatically when one parent lost a job, business was slow, or unexpected costs arose. And I found that food's meaning to middle-class parents could shift in lockstep with these financial changes. Overnight, food could go from being a teaching tool to a means of compensating for tougher circumstances. That is, how parents used food was extremely sensitive to whether they were making ends meet. When things were going well, parents could focus on food as a medium for teaching kids about nutrition. When things got tough, these same parents could turn to food as an antidote for hardship.

Alvaro and Sofia Morales, parents of three, showed me just how intensely food's meaning could vacillate *within* a family. As we sat in the Moraleses' living room one evening, Alvaro explained that a few months ago, he and his family had been eating very nutritiously. But in January, Alvaro had been laid off from his job in construction management, an unexpected loss that shook his self-esteem and his family's world. When Alvaro was gainfully employed, feeding his family had felt like relatively smooth sailing. But now, things were different.

"We used to be really conscious about clean food," Sofia said, putting her hand on Alvaro's knee as they sat side by side on a gray sofa. "The big shift was when we started having all of this financial stress and all this burden—we became so focused on just *surviving*."

Sofia's mention of survival took me back to an afternoon on Nyah's couch. "I'm just trying to survive," Nyah had told me. She hadn't been thinking ahead. She had been trying to move through each moment in time, to get by until her prospects improved. Certainly, the Moraleses were in better financial shape than Nyah had been, but their mentalities had striking parallels.

"Now we're just in survival mode." Alvaro echoed his wife, gently placing his hand atop hers. Alvaro rattled off all the expenses currently weighing on them: their eldest daughter's college tuition next year, their son's soccer club, their youngest daughter's day care, and Sofia's emergency root canal that their dental insurance wouldn't cover.

"It's just so overwhelming." Alvaro sighed, his brown eyes widening.

Food was also overwhelming them. What had once been Alvaro's well of joy had become a major source of angst. Before losing his job, Alvaro had reveled in weekends spent grocery shopping. The kids would pile into the minivan with their dad and he'd hit all of his favorite stores. Their first stop was Whole Foods, where they'd grab fresh, seasonal fruit and specialty items like cured olives and goat's-milk yogurt. Then they'd head over to their local deli for the best cuts of meat. They'd end up at the farmers' market, where Alvaro would choose vegetables for the week and his kids would sneak as many free samples as they could. But now, because of all of the other stresses his family was facing, food was often the last thing on Alvaro's mind.

"To eat healthy," Alvaro told me, "it takes more resources."

Because Alvaro's resources were now in short supply, his weekend shopping itinerary looked different. There was no more perusing the aisles at Whole Foods or sampling peaches at the market. "Now it's just 'What's on sale at Safeway and kind of organic?'" Alvaro chuckled, though I could tell he didn't really find it funny. "We're still trying to keep the same frame set, but we don't have the luxuries, so sometimes we have to buy the ninety-nine-cent chicken and it's just got to stretch a little bit longer. Maybe make two meals out of it instead of four-ninety-nine-a-pound chicken that's gonna be for one meal."

Even though Alvaro still cared about what his kids ate, he found it hard to care as much when he knew that he had less to devote to their diets. Comparing how they used to eat with their current consumption stung. Alvaro still strove to teach his kids about nutrition and health, but he also found himself using food to compensate for the stress that his job loss had inflicted on his family.

"Sometimes I just can't pull it together," he said, closing his eyes for a moment. "And that's when we end up picking up fast food." Alvaro didn't love fast food—he questioned the quality of the meat—but the kids did. And these days, his family needed any morale boost they could get.

Alvaro and Sofia weren't alone in struggling with the dietary challenges that came with shifting finances. Chastity Banks similarly felt that she was being stretched too thin. I first met Chastity one Saturday afternoon at Target. Chastity had caught my attention when I spotted her with her three daughters in the cereal aisle. I was awestruck watching Chastity as she absorbed the two younger daughters' pleas with a seemingly endless well of patience. Even as the youngest—who was seven—tugged on the bottom of her shirt and whined for her attention, Chastity acted remarkably, almost eerily, calm. I was so amazed by Chastity's poise that I asked her for an interview. *Maybe I can uncover the secret to her serenity,* I thought.

But I soon learned that internally, Chastity, like most moms, was battling feelings of inadequacy. With these emotions compounded by a recent financial loss, she felt stretched to the brink and unable to focus on her daughters' diets the way she wanted.

"I'm concerned about their health and what they're eating," Chastity told me the next weekend over two cups of jasmine tea at a bookstore café. Chastity's wiry black hair was pulled back in a bun, and she blew on her steaming tea as we spoke.

A year prior, Chastity's husband, James, had decided to go back to school to become a chef. The decision had not been reached easily; it had been the culmination of countless late-night discussions that unfolded around the kitchen table as Chastity repeatedly plugged the numbers—her income, James's income, school tuition, the girls' extracurriculars—into her phone's calculator. After what seemed like the hundredth calculation, Chastity saw a way forward. She understood the kinds of financial tweaks they'd have to make to pull it off.

In the long run, a culinary school degree and new career as a chef would leave James more fulfilled and boost the Bankses' overall household income. But in the short term, the transition set the family back financially. James continued working the night shift for the postal service, but he went down from full-time to part-time hours. James's salary reduction hadn't hit the Bankses hard enough to qualify them for federal food assistance. But the change had placed an enormous amount of stress on Chastity, who, overnight, had become her family's primary breadwinner. Chastity started picking up more hours at the hospital where she worked as a medical technician. She went from spending mornings and evenings with her kids to showing them how to use the defrost function on the microwave.

"I don't want to disappoint." Chastity paused. "And I feel like I'm disappointing them."

Chastity's biggest challenge came from not being home. All the extra hours at work meant less time to grocery shop and cook for her kids the way they'd come to expect over the years. It meant less time with her kids overall. "I feel bad." Chastity sighed. "It's kind of a struggle because I did stay at home with them for a little while and so they kind of got used to that. But now it's like, I can't do that anymore."

Her lack of time was especially challenging in the mornings. Chastity wanted her thirteen-year-old and seven-year-old to eat a healthy and satiating breakfast before school. This was essential for their education. Brain food, Chastity called it. But Chastity was rarely home when they were getting ready for school. What could the girls eat when both she and her husband were gone?

"I don't want them touching the oven or the stove," Chastity said. "I don't want a fire or someone to get hurt. So I try to buy little oranges, like the Cuties." The kids sometimes ate those for breakfast. They also had Pop-Tarts and granola bars around for something quick. This was fine, Chastity felt, but it didn't make her feel great.

"It's rough," Chastity said. "Nothing's as healthy as cooking your food and having a good hearty breakfast, huh?"

With both her and James out of the house most of the day, Chastity also didn't want her kids to feel neglected. She wanted them to know, deep down, that she still cared about what they wanted, food included. That's why, rather than saying no all the time, Chastity negotiated with them. "It's a lot of back-and-forth. It's give-and-take." She chuckled. "But maybe lately more of a give, rather than me taking." Chastity bought small plastic bins that she labeled with each of her daughters' names and filled with snacks for them to eat when she wasn't home. Each morning before leaving for work, she'd ensure that the bins had fruit snacks, juice boxes, Fig Newtons, and oatmeal packets in them. On her evening drive home from work, Chastity would swing by a nearby Burger King to grab a carton of fries. Those fries would tide her kids over while she put dinner together. Chastity would toss a bag of vegetables in the microwave to steam and spread frozen tater tots across a tray to bake in the oven.

It wasn't that Chastity wanted her kids' diets to tip toward the processed end. But amid all of the chaos in their lives currently, it actually felt good to give in a little. It felt easier to nod in agreement than shake her head and fight. Doing so, I realized, helped Chastity stay as calm as she appeared. It helped her have energy for the extra twenty hours a week she was putting in at the hospital. For Chastity, food could help bridge gaps.

But when Chastity had the time—when she worked a late instead of an early-morning shift—she made sure that she cooked the girls a special meal. "I'll make a full breakfast," Chastity said, setting her hands on the table. "I'll make biscuit sandwiches like they have at McDonald's, with the sausage."

Even though Chastity knew sausage biscuits weren't the healthiest, cooking something healthy wasn't what these mornings were about anymore. Amid the tougher circumstances the Bankses were currently weathering, these mornings were about Chastity's love of her family and quality time together. They were about showing herself and her kids that she was there for them.

Chastity took menu requests from the girls. She picked up the bacon and waffles they asked for to show them that even though she was not around as much, she still cared deeply about them, about their wants and their needs. The mornings Chastity worked, while she sterilized ultrasound equipment or collected specimens from the lab, she thought of her daughters lined up at the dining-room table. She pictured their smiles and the sound of them chomping on waffles, their front teeth coated in warm maple syrup.

One day, Chastity hoped, she and James would settle into a new family routine. James would finish school and start earning a real income again. Chastity would scale back her hours at the hospital; she'd be home in the mornings to take the kids to school. In the afternoons, she'd pick them up again and get home early enough to make dinner. Maybe, she mused, James would even use his newfound culinary skills to help get an evening meal on the table. In this distant future, Chastity thought, food would get easier again.

CHAPTER 15

Becoming American

It was a warm September afternoon when I first met Teresa Lopez. The two of us sat at two desks in an empty social studies classroom at Lincoln High School, where her only son, Esteban, was in the ninth grade. A thin ray of sun streamed through an open window, hitting a recently cleaned green chalkboard. Teresa's curly brown hair was pulled back in a taut bun, and she wore bright pink lipstick, a floral top, and boot-cut jeans. Around her neck hung a pearl necklace with a silver cross, and over her shoulder a tote bag with the words SAN FRANCISCO in cursive.

Born in Sinaloa, Mexico, Teresa had immigrated to the United States sixteen years ago, first to Los Angeles and later, after separating from her husband, up to the Bay Area. "Since then, I have been here," Teresa said softly, "facing a thousand different hurdles to get ahead in life."

Over the years, Teresa had worked hard to come to terms with the realities of her situation. It was a life harder, in many ways, than the one she'd led before crossing the border. Since arriving in the U.S., Teresa had survived domestic abuse and a contentious separation. She'd cleaned toilets and nannied rich people's kids. She'd been laid off and evicted. She'd lived in her van. She'd wiped away Esteban's tears when she couldn't afford to get him even the cheapest television set.

But, Teresa told me, things had grown easier over time. It's not that her life improved. Rather, she had, bit by bit, come to terms with everything. Teresa had worked to reconcile the differences between her expectations and her reality. She had fought to center gratitude over disappointment.

"Little by little, one forgets about what was left there, what is over there." Teresa sighed, thinking of the village where she'd spent the first twenty years of her life. "It has been difficult, but little by little one overcomes it. One learns to live with what happens."

Over the past few years, Teresa had worked full-time as a house cleaner. She always made rent, but her paychecks' timing often meant that there were certain days each month when she didn't have money to restock the kitchen. The cupboards, normally piled high with flour tortillas, black beans, and canned vegetables, were bare. A few white onions rolled around the vegetable drawer, rather than the usual zucchini, squash, and heads of broccoli.

"If I don't have anything when it is the first few days of the month," Teresa said, "I have to pay rent, insurance, such and such. I tell Esteban, 'Let's go experiment, come on! Let's see what we can come up with.'" Teresa smiled, her dark eyes crinkling at the corners as she described spinning hardship into opportunity. "Sometimes when there isn't anything, you need to invent something out of what you already have."

Hard as being an inventor was, Teresa believed that the sacrifices she had made to come to America—and to survive in America—would yield Esteban a better life. Here, he had opportunities unthinkable south of the border. Teresa was undocumented, but Esteban's American citizenship was his ticket. His future was brighter than hers—he would speak fluent English, go to college, and get a good job with benefits. He wouldn't have to worry like she had. He wouldn't have to give up the things she had given up.

To secure Esteban's future, Teresa kept putting one foot in

front of the other. She scrubbed more toilets. She babysat on the weekends, bringing Esteban with her to help watch the children. She learned enough English to help her son with his social studies homework. She attended parent-teacher conferences and back-to-school nights. She joined a Hispanic parent association at Esteban's school, building a support network with other parents whom she could rely on to look out for her and her son. Sometimes, this country still felt as foreign to Teresa as the day she'd first stepped foot on its soil. But, she told herself, Esteban's future was worth it.

One of four siblings, Teresa was raised in a village by a mom who worked and a grandma who cooked for their extended family. Teresa remembered running home from school in the early afternoon for midday *comida* to find *caldos* or *sopas de fideo*. No meal was complete unless all nine kids—Teresa, her siblings, and her cousins—were seated around the kitchen table. "We were the typical family." Teresa smiled. "Home-centered, home-cooked meals." No one ever ate alone, and there was always enough for everyone. "My mother would say, 'Where one eats, three eat. Where three eat, six eat.'"

Still, there was little money to pull together grand, elaborate meals. Sometimes, she and the other kids ate beans and rice for days in a row. They would complain, begging for something else. "In this house," her grandmother would reply, "you eat what we have. This is not a buffet, nor is this a restaurant. We are all going to eat the same thing." Teresa glanced out the open window. "And all of us, whether we liked it or not, ate it."

Today, Teresa's greatest joy came from preparing the Sinaloan foods of her childhood for Esteban. While they too sometimes had to scrape by on rice and beans for a few days, more often she got to revel in watching him devour her tostadas, *tamales de camarón*, and *sopes*. Esteban never felt shortchanged flavor-wise by his mom. "You're always inventing dishes, and they come out good," he complimented her.

The longer Teresa spent in America, the more she saw how this country was changing her. She was starting, slowly, almost imperceptibly, to experience what had once seemed impossible. She felt more and more American.

"I feel that here is my home," Teresa explained, "and that this country is more so my country than over there." She waved her arm as if pointing toward Mexico.

Esteban's Americanness hit Teresa even harder. All his life, Esteban had attended American schools. He'd made American friends with names like Clint and Logan. He'd played American sports like football and watched American TV programs in English like *Sesame Street*. His diet was more American too. As much as Esteban devoured his mom's tamales and *aguachile*, he also loved Kraft mac and cheese and Krispy Kreme doughnuts. Teresa, too, ate those foods with a smile on her face.

Scholars call what Teresa and Esteban were doing *acculturation,* or the process by which immigrants begin to adopt aspects of American culture, including certain ideologies, beliefs, and practices. And they call the Americanization of Teresa's and Esteban's diets *dietary acculturation,* or the process by which immigrants start to adopt the dietary practices of the countries they settle in. Dietary acculturation, it's argued, is a big way that immigrants assimilate into American society. As they eat American food, they *become* American.

Nutritionally, dietary acculturation in America has its downsides; in general, the more immigrants and their children adopt American dietary habits, the lower quality their diets become. This is largely because America's highly commercialized, relatively cheap, and generally unhealthy food landscape creates new opportunities for consumption. Immigrant families start dining out and carrying out more and eating greater amounts of convenience foods, sugar-sweetened beverages, and red meat.[1] What this means is that as these families adopt more features of the American diet, they may actually be *worse off* nutritionally.

Immigrant parents are usually deemed responsible for their kids' dietary acculturation. Supposedly, kids' diets are Americanizing under their parents' direct supervision, making parents the ones to blame for declines in kids' nutrition. But this narrative oversimplifies the situation.

Teresa didn't always see what Esteban was eating. In fact, Esteban spent quite a lot of time away from his mom. In the school cafeteria, he ate shrink-wrapped hot dogs and defrosted sweet potato fries. When he hung out with friends on Sundays after church, they spent their last bills at 7-Eleven and Sonic. On weekday afternoons, as he awaited Teresa's return from work in their one-bedroom, second-story apartment, he watched commercials for Cocoa Puffs and Mountain Dew flash across the screen. During those times, Teresa had at best a sense of—but rarely a hand in—the American foods Esteban filled his stomach with.

Other times, though, Teresa herself helped Americanize Esteban's diet. While Teresa still cooked most evenings, she downshifted her family's consumption of traditional Sinaloan foods. She and Esteban ate more convenience foods, more meat, and more fast food than she had growing up. In the supermarket, Esteban grabbed boxes of Froot Loops and cans of Cheez Whiz off the shelves, negotiating with his mom to give them a chance. "For fun!" he'd joke, and Teresa would laugh, pretending not to notice as he tossed them in the cart. Other nights, Esteban would beg his mom for a McDonald's cheeseburger and fries. If it was also her payday, she'd oblige.

Why did Teresa do that? I wondered.

In public discourse, commentators have posed similar questions, usually judgmentally. Why do immigrant parents incorporate American food into their kids' diets? they ask. Why don't these parents do more to keep their kids' diets healthy when they come to America? Why don't these parents work harder to feed their kids healthier traditional foods and protect them from unhealthy American ones?

These questions are deeply problematic. For one, they insidiously shift the blame away from America's unhealthy food environment and onto the parents. They present a structural problem as an individual one for which parents alone are culpable. But a bigger issue with these questions, I realized, was their underlying flawed assumption. They assumed that immigrant parents *saw* American food as unhealthy or worse for their kids but chose it anyway.

But what if, I wondered, the opposite was true? What if immigrant moms actually regarded aspects of American food as *better*? What if they saw partially Americanizing their kids' diets as a *good thing* rather than a problem? What if, when moms fed their kids both traditional and American foods, they were actually trying to do *right* by them?

Teresa said yes to Esteban's food requests, in many ways, for the same reasons other low-income parents obliged. The Froot Loops and the Cheez Whiz offered Teresa an opportunity, amid scarcity, to emotionally nourish Esteban. Teresa's financial scarcity could also force her prioritization away from Esteban's nutritional intake, making a Tuesday-night McDonald's run a reasonable choice for her family.

But there was more to it than that. Immigrant moms like Teresa also faced a deeper cultural tension that left them caught between the foods of their home country and the foods of this new one. Teresa worked to preserve the meaningful culinary traditions that anchored her to her childhood and extended family. Even if Esteban had never lived in Mexico himself, Teresa wanted him to feel a sense of belonging and rootedness to his homeland.

Because of this, Esteban's adoration of his mom's cooking

filled Teresa with an immense satisfaction. To watch him devour her dishes—the same dishes she'd devoured as a girl at her grandmother's wooden table—made Teresa feel connected to her family thousands of miles away. Sometimes, that food was all she had to remind her—the last vestige of a culture she was now alone tasked with keeping alive for her son. She wanted her son to remember that he was Mexican as well as American. When she prepared traditional Sinaloan dishes for him, Teresa showed Esteban that. She remembered who she was too. Teresa had given up so much to come to the U.S. At the very least, she didn't have to sacrifice their identity.

Teresa also clung to Sinaloan food because it helped her survive America. For Teresa, getting by in this country meant continually overcoming the daily realities of living undocumented. Getting paid under the table meant perpetual insecurity. She had no benefits and no recourse if things went sour. Living without papers meant that Teresa had to both accept and simultaneously try to forget that at any second, she could be deported. She knew that every moment with her son could also be her last, even as she prayed that, God willing, it would never come to that.

As these hardships wore Teresa down, it was often food that could help pick her back up. Teresa savored the comfort that came from cooking the same dishes she'd grown up with. These were the dishes she knew like the back of her hand, the ones that smelled and tasted like her grandmother's kitchen. When life in America yet again proved far more trying than Teresa could have ever imagined, that food was her and Esteban's cushion. Even after an arduous day scrubbing floors, she could catch up with Esteban over her grandmother's *chilorio*. When language barriers prevented her from helping her son with his science homework, she could bring him a warm cup of milk with *pan dulce* for extra motivation. No matter what, Teresa could nourish herself and her son with Sinaloan foods.

Yet moms like Teresa also had to reckon with the reality that their kids' tastes—not to mention their own—were changing in the midst of their immigration story. Esteban didn't always want the foods Teresa prepared. Sometimes, he just wanted the stuff he saw his friends at school eat. He wanted to fit in, not stand out. One morning, he felt embarrassed bringing a thermos of Teresa's soup to school, and he begged her to make him a peanut butter and jelly sandwich instead. Pleas like these could make Teresa's heart sink. It's not that she disapproved of PB and J; she just felt rejected. *Who was this child she was raising?* she asked herself. How quickly he had forgotten where he came from. How little he seemed to understand the sacrifices his mom had made to get him here.

And yet Teresa also saw where her son was coming from. She knew that part of Esteban's future success in this country hinged on being American. He would never make it here if he didn't learn its cultural practices, expectations, and norms. Food was a part of that. He needed to eat American food to fit in. As his mother, she had a duty to help him with that. It was her job to make sure he succeeded here.

Because of this, Teresa didn't regard Esteban's diet as an either/or trade-off. She didn't believe that he needed to eat *only* Mexican or *only* American food; there was space for both the traditional and the new. Esteban could eat Teresa's soups one day and a turkey sandwich the next. "I pick up on the good things here and conserve the good parts of my culture," Teresa said, interlocking her fingers. "The two are united."

The point is, some immigrant moms, like Teresa, did not fear the Americanization of their kids' diets. Rather, they saw it in some ways as a positive. While still working to hold tight to certain dietary traditions, moms also embraced the opportunity to eat and feed their kids coveted foods newly available to them in the U.S. Even though they recognized that at times, doing so came at a nutritional expense, it was also worth it. The symbolic victory of feeding kids American foods often outweighed the costs because it achieved multiple goals at once: it buffered their children and boosted their own maternal self-worth. It helped kids fit in culturally, to feel a sense of belonging and rootedness that moms themselves could struggle to secure.

Teresa believed that Esteban benefited from eating in America. She saw the benefits for herself too. Teresa explained to me, a wide grin on her face, that when it came to food, "I am learning from him." After enrolling in a nutrition course at school, Esteban had taught Teresa about healthy sources of protein and the difference between organic and conventionally grown produce. He had shown her YouTube cooking channels. When they grocery shopped, he pointed out different kinds of fish she'd never heard about. All of the milk and meat he was eating here, Teresa was also convinced, was helping her son grow taller than his cousins in Mexico. More than that, Esteban was helping Teresa and himself fit into American society, educating them about their food choices and bringing some highly welcome diversity into their diets.

For Teresa, the personal symbolic victory of American food was powerful. American dining became the bright spot, the happy ending (even though it was ongoing) of an otherwise difficult immigration story. Being able to buy her son American food offered Teresa momentary proof that she had made it, that the seemingly endless hardships she'd endured were worth it and that she had done better for her son. On the evenings when she could get her son to eat something satisfying and satiating, Teresa also felt the optimism she'd brought to the States swell up inside of her. They were poor, yes, but they could still afford to try the deep-dish pizza down the street. They could still split a basket of chicken fingers and sweet potato fries. When Teresa looked back on how hard things had been those first few years in this country, she knew things were better now. The future, too, was bright.

Teresa remembered herself as a lanky girl begging her grandmother for sugary cereals. Now here she was, able to buy Esteban a box of Froot Loops. She recalled strolling by a sit-down restaurant on her walk home from elementary school, peering in longingly to see families gathered around white tablecloths, sharing dishes she knew her family could never afford. Now she took Esteban to Red Robin for his birthday, the two of them cozied into a corner booth, sipping their Pepsis out of tall glasses and joking about their ornery landlord. When things were rough, Teresa reminded herself of how lucky she was and how hard she'd worked to raise Esteban in a country where she could delight him, every so often, with delicious foods and unique flavors. She had sacrificed so he could have better. And in those moments, Teresa thought, maybe she'd succeeded. Maybe, after all—and despite how it often felt—she was winning.

PART IV

Emotion

I learned to make my mind large, as the universe is large,
so that there is room for paradoxes.
— MAXINE HONG KINGSTON, *THE WOMAN WARRIOR*

CHAPTER 16

Downscaling

I first met Brenda Rojas on an overcast afternoon inside her son's tae kwon do studio. The studio was one storefront among many in a vast, bustling strip mall. Brenda and her daughter, Ava, sat in a waiting area. Spotting me from afar, Brenda waved gregariously as I weaved through a crowd of families to join them. At five feet two inches with short, curly hair, copper skin, and the same thin-framed glasses as her daughter, Brenda was as cheery as her bright pink lipstick. But her torn jeans and frayed sweater hinted at a harder reality.

Amid the sounds of children counting out sit-ups, shouting, and smacking assorted pads, the studio was noisy. Brenda suggested we head next door to Burger King to chat. Inside, I treated each of us to a cup of coffee. "Two Splendas and two creams," she told the cashier. While we waited for our drinks, Brenda entertained me with stories from her job as a sales associate in the gardening section of a large hardware store. Wandering through aisles of plants all day, Brenda said with a chuckle, made her feel like she worked in a jungle.

While I was struck by Brenda's positivity, a few minutes into our conversation, it became clear that Brenda's story was nowhere near as sunny as her disposition. Over the past two decades, she'd experienced deportation, family separation, unemployment, and poverty.

Brenda had been born in the United States and moved to

Colombia at the age of five. As a teenager, she had married and quickly thereafter given birth to Ava. Unfortunately, when Brenda tried to return to the U.S. with her daughter in tow, there was a mix-up with Ava's documents.

"The papers for my daughter were lost," she explained, slowly stirring the cream into her coffee. Ava stayed in Colombia with her father, Victor, and her grandparents while Brenda moved north to start working and sending remittances. Alone in an unfamiliar country, Brenda soon encountered a new source of despair. In 2001, she learned that she had type 2 diabetes. The unexpected diagnosis traumatized her.

"Psychologically, I was alone," Brenda said, her face hardening as she recalled the feelings of hopelessness. "I was separated from my child and my husband. When they say to me I have diabetes, I feel like I was going to die because no one explained to you in a good way… they say, 'Oh, you have diabetes, it's this and that.' I say, 'Okay.' I went home. I was crying. I went to sleep."

Thankfully, Brenda was not alone for long. Victor came to the United States a year later, but Brenda would have to wait four more years to reunite with her daughter. During that time, she and Victor lived paycheck to paycheck, constantly relocating from one apartment to another amid an unforgiving cycle of unemployment and reemployment. Every eight to ten months, one of them lost a job, whether it was her husband's position as a night janitor or hers as a cashier at Jack in the Box.

In 2008, Brenda was finally able to bring ten-year-old Ava to the United States and discovered soon after that she was pregnant with a second child, a son they would name Rodrigo. With a baby on the way, Brenda was grateful to land a job at a video store a block from their apartment. "I work at that video store for eight years," she told me. "But then the video store closed because people don't rent any more videos. They watch it on their computer. And then I was without job for almost a year."

The lack of job security made caring for her own health and

that of her family difficult. Brenda learned to manage her diabetes using whatever means were available at any given moment. Occasionally she got health insurance through work, which gave her access to oral medications and insulin injections. Most of the time, she received no treatment at all. After one unexpected layoff, Brenda found under-the-table work at her son's elementary school and used the money to manage her condition.

"The principal of the elementary gave me a job—a special job. I'm not going to say." She smiled slightly. "He gave me like twenty hours a week. He gave me good hours to pay my medicine."

Yet for all of Brenda's struggles—financial, legal, and health-related—she exuded an unmistakable air of appreciation. There was more hope and gratitude in her tone than despondency. After mistaking her original diabetes diagnosis for a death sentence, Brenda rejoiced when she learned her condition wasn't fatal. The morning after being diagnosed, Brenda got out of bed. "When I woke up, I was like, I am still alive, I didn't die! I thought I was going to die that night. I thought I wasn't going to see my children, my husband. I woke up and I was like, thank you!" Brenda continued, "Every day that I wake up, I have to smile. I am still alive."

Brenda's positive attitude, while heartening, was also a bit perplexing. At the time we met, Brenda worried that she and her family were just one paycheck away from eviction. *One* paycheck. She couldn't have been living any closer to the bone, and her situation was far from unusual. Over half of the low-income families I met, like millions of Americans every year, had experienced a forced move or eviction. Sociologists like Matthew Desmond have shown that this kind of housing instability is all too common, with around 15 percent of children born in major U.S. cities experiencing an eviction by age fifteen. These kinds of forced moves have concrete negative impacts on families. They increase families' financial stress and material hardship. They fuel parental stress and moms' depression. They increase the chances of kids experiencing food insecurity. They strip away the psychological and physical security of having a home.[1]

Eviction was top of mind for Brenda these days because she had just gone through it eighteen months prior, after her landlord had unexpectedly raised the rent. With Victor hunting for work, they started falling behind on rent each month. After three months, her landlord got fed up, and the Rojases ended up on the street. After two weeks in a shelter and then two months on friends' couches, the Rojas family finally moved into their own apartment. There, the stove worked, the water was hot, and all the doors locked. The kids were able to stay in the same public school. For a moment, Brenda could breathe.

But now, because Brenda's boss had recently reduced her hours at the gardening center, she foresaw them barely making their rent this month. If they came up short, they'd soon be hunting for a new place.

And yet, Brenda didn't behave like disaster was imminent. How, I wondered, could Brenda act so thankful when there was so much ongoing struggle and uncertainty in her life? The life Brenda lived in San Jose seemed to diverge so drastically from what she had expected when she stepped foot on American soil years before. So then why did Brenda seem okay with—even thankful for—this reality?

Brenda wasn't the only low-income mom I met who continually highlighted the positive while recounting the tremendous material hardships, struggles, and anxieties she lived with. Over time, I learned that this glass-half-full outlook wasn't something that necessarily came naturally to these moms. It wasn't that Brenda just happened to be inherently optimistic or prone to seeing the brighter side of things. These mothers' optimism was, in fact, a survival strategy—a tool for resilience in the midst of adversity. And it had serious implications for how they approached their kids' diets.

A few months into my research, I began to grapple with a contradiction. I walked away from interviews with moms like Brenda knowing that they were parenting under exceptionally challenging conditions that made feeding kids difficult. But overall, these moms didn't seem all too worried about their kids' diets. Sure, they talked about wanting their kids to eat healthy and they voiced frustration about how that didn't always happen. But they still seemed, somewhat surprisingly, optimistic about how their kids ate.

I knew it wasn't that simple. I came to see that these moms' emphasis on the positive was a coping mechanism they employed in order to resolve the tension between their aspirations and their realities. Like Brenda, most low-income moms dealt with enormous challenges, be it securing affordable housing or quality health insurance. There were obstacles that Brenda wished she could resolve; she wished she could ensure that she and Victor had steady wages that let them put money in savings and that landlords would stop raising the rent each year. But when it came to those kinds of big changes—the things that could really turn things around for families—moms like Brenda told me they felt resigned. They knew that these weren't the kinds of changes they could expect to see anytime soon.

So, with limited chances to make things materially better for themselves and their children, moms fought to *feel* better about how things were, to accept their current realities rather than constantly wishing for better ones. They took this fight on *internally,* trying to change how they felt inside. Sociologists call this *emotion work,* a term introduced in 1979 by the sociologist Arlie Hochschild.[2] As the name implies, emotion work is the work people do to manipulate their own emotions—monitoring, inhibiting, evoking, and shaping them in different ways—so that their feelings are in line with what they think they should feel or what they want to feel. Emotion work involves more than just displaying the right emotions on the outside. It means trying to conjure up the appropriate feelings through managing the ones that naturally emerge.

People engage in emotion work for a number of reasons. A major one is that it's often far easier to change one's thoughts about one's reality than to alter reality itself. I may not be able to move into a new house, but I can work to change the way I feel about my current house. I may lose my job, but I can convince myself that I never really liked that job anyway. We all do emotion work. And we're told it's a good thing; self-help blogs and articles that advise us to change our mindsets, practice gratitude, and focus on life's blessings reinforce the idea that we can make ourselves happy despite our surroundings.

Like foodwork, emotion work within families is largely gendered. Moms are widely seen as responsible for helping mediate and manage family members' emotions to keep family life harmonious and households running smoothly. These goals are also achieved when moms work on their *own* emotions. When Renata tried to find the humor in José's penchant for fast food, for instance, she worked on her emotions to transform frustration into amusement.

Discussions of nutritional inequality rarely, if ever, mention emotions or emotion work. But I learned that emotions have a lot to do with how families eat. As I watched moms across income levels managing their emotions, I came to understand how broader inequalities burrowed themselves deep inside of moms, shaping the thoughts and feelings they used to get by from day to day. And these thoughts and feelings had everything to do with how moms then approached food with their kids.

As I'll explain in the next chapter, privileged moms engaged in emotion-work strategies that helped pull their families farther away from the middle and bottom; these moms strove to manage their feelings of anxiety through doing more. They shopped more, cooked more, and monitored more. They worked harder to get their children the best food they possibly could, devoting extraordinary financial, temporal, and emotional resources to constantly improve upon and refine their kids' tastes and diets. Their work never felt complete, so they kept searching for new and better ways of eating. In this manner, affluent moms' emotion-work strategies catapulted their families even further away from families with fewer resources.

By contrast, low-income moms' strategies to deal with unjust, challenging circumstances worked in the opposite direction. For moms like Brenda, moms for whom real, meaningful improvements in their circumstances were rarely attainable, there was a sense of resignation that their kids' diets might never be what they hoped. This is not to say that these moms stopped trying to get their kids to eat healthy food. Many still did what they could. But they knew the deck was stacked against them. Rather than fighting an uphill battle they'd likely ultimately lose, they worked to see their kids' diets' virtues rather than fixating on their shortcomings. They worked to appreciate what they had rather than desiring what they lacked. They found a survival strategy that let them feed, eat, and preserve their dignity. But this strategy could also inadvertently cement less privileged families' diets in place by lowering moms' expectations and beliefs in what was possible food-wise.

Low-income moms' survival strategy involved a particular kind of emotion work, what the sociologist Marianne Cooper calls *downscaling*.[3] Downscaling is when people lower their expectations to adapt to and survive a difficult life. The low-income moms I met downscaled their expectations about almost everything, whether it was their job prospects, financial futures, or the food their families ate. Downscaling provided an approach for navigating persistent hardships, an approach that had profound implications for their kids' diets.

I met Lorena Garcia, a single mom of four and grandmother of two, at a coffee shop one November afternoon. She arrived with her sixteen-year-old daughter, Linda, and Linda's six-month-old son.

Lorena, a short, stocky woman with wavy brown hair and choppy bangs, spent hours talking with me about how she loved incorporating her mixed Mexican and Filipina heritage into her cooking. To Lorena, eating healthy meant consuming "more of the good foods, like eating fruits and vegetables. Trying not to snack on garbage so much. That kind of stuff. That's what I think healthy is."

Lorena felt her family was falling short of her dietary aspirations. In addition to her own sweet tooth and proclivity for McDonald's, she was frustrated by her kids' lack of interest in fruits and nuts. Her kids pleaded for flaky, salty treats that dissolved in their mouths but never filled them up. Linda, Lorena said, letting out a tired sigh, had a "chip problem." Lorena also mentioned several other barriers her family faced when it came to healthy eating, including her recent job loss and subsequent lack of reliable income and the fact that when she was employed, she was generally working sixty or more hours a week and barely had time to grocery shop, let alone cook.

But when I asked Lorena directly if she faced any challenges when it came to food, her answer caught me off guard. She insisted that no, she actually didn't have any challenges at all.

What is she talking about? I wondered. Minutes earlier, Lorena had detailed a number of serious issues, job insecurity and time scarcity among them. Her response didn't make any sense until weeks later when, replaying the audio recording of our conversation, I realized that Lorena had interpreted the question differently than I'd intended. She was thinking about challenges in relative terms, comparing her current situation to previous periods in her life. When she stacked this current moment up against earlier, more difficult ones, there was hardly anything challenging about food today.

"I don't really have any challenges at this time," Lorena had said, taking a sip of coffee and allowing her mind to wander back to her kids' early years. "There was a time in our lives where—before I even met my husband—my children and I had it really bad. I had barely enough to pay the bills and not much to pay for food."

Even though Lorena had applied for Section 8 housing, she was thousands down on a never-ending waiting list. Like many low-income moms, she turned to an unaffordable and unforgiving private housing market that continually jostled her around. There was a three-year period during which Lorena moved six times. Once, her landlady kicked her out after she was four hundred dollars short on rent two months in a row. Another time, she initiated the move after discovering mold in her kids' room. She could tolerate maggots in the sink, but the mold was too much. They'd moved into a new apartment, only to discover a family of rats living between the bathroom and bedroom walls. As much as Lorena hated the never-ending moves, she didn't see much choice. She did every move alone, her toddler and baby in tow.

Moving so much made everything else virtually impossible. Keeping her job as a sales associate at Old Navy was difficult. Lorena relied on her aunt to watch the kids when she worked, but sometimes her aunt was unavailable, and Lorena had to bring the kids with her to the store. When she wasn't working, she was using up gas driving around in search of better housing. She was earning just above California's minimum wage—at the time, nine dollars an hour—which meant Lorena could generally come up with the first month's rent on a new place. But she almost never had enough to put a security deposit down if a landlord asked for one. That security deposit was her diaper supply for the next month. There were no savings. There was no buffer. There was just getting through each day and praying the next one would be easier.

Compared to back then, food today wasn't too challenging for Lorena. For one, she could regularly buy it. Now her kids always had enough to eat. She, too, generally ate enough. Sure, Lorena was frustrated that food was pricey, that she rarely had time to cook, and that her kids only wanted junk. But Lorena could also shine a positive light on all of those things. Sure, food was expensive—but at least she had enough to scrape by. Sure, she rarely had time to cook—but at least she lived near a Jack in the Box. And sure, her kids only wanted Lay's potato chips and Dr Pepper—but at least she could afford to get them exactly what they liked.

Even in the face of hardship, Lorena was resilient. Part of that resilience stemmed from her tremendous ability to reconcile her reality with her ideal; by thinking back to times when things were really tough, Lorena could downscale her emotions into feeling better about any current shortcomings.

When things were hard, other low-income parents focused not only on the past but also on the future. They concentrated on the temporariness of it all, and they shared hope for a new day. Nyah, for instance, often assured herself—and me—that better times lay right ahead. As much as Nyah's attention was often on daily survival, she also worked to orient her gaze toward a hopeful future. "It's just not our year," she told me one morning as we drove to the drugstore. "It'll get better when my health gets better."

Turning left into the parking lot, Nyah sighed. "I'm not gonna be down forever."

"Watch this!" Paige shouted. She did an effortless backbend that looked as if she had a rubber hose for a spine. On a Monday evening, I sat in Dana's living room with Madison sidled up beside me on the worn beige couch. While the muted TV played in the background, Madison and I cheered Paige on as she performed her latest gymnastics routine, flipping and spinning with endless energy. Dana was cleaning up from dinner in the kitchen, occasionally popping her head into the living room to check on us.

I thought back to the first time Dana and I had met. In our initial conversation, Dana had explained that her family's diet had been unusual lately. "This week has been so busy," she told me, twirling the silver chain hanging around her neck. "We got deli sandwiches on Saturday, because we were painting and dizzy. It is out of the ordinary. Then we went to sushi dinner, which was kind of cheating." Dana paused. "This weekend doesn't count for food."

More recently, Dana and I had taken her daughters out to an early Friday dinner at a local taqueria. Families, twenty-something couples, and hordes of teenagers were packed within its four bright orange walls. We lined up to order at the counter. When both Madison and Paige ordered soda, Dana quickly pointed out that they didn't normally do that. "It's Friday," she said with a laugh, handing the cashier the dollar bills.

To an outsider, it may have seemed like Dana didn't really care about her kids' diets the way she said she did. But I knew it was more complicated than that. Dana was genuinely concerned about the soda. She knew it was bad for the girls' teeth and loaded with sugar that drove their hyperactivity late into the evening.

In a less immediately challenging world, Dana would have had the bandwidth to politely inform the cashier that, actually, her girls would be drinking water this evening. Dana would have then explained to Madison and Paige that soda had too much added sugar and artificial coloring, and that it would give them cavities. Water, she would've assured them, was a better choice for them, tonight and every night. Next, she would have stood patiently—calmly, even—as Paige spiraled into a tantrum, throwing her sparkly necklace on the floor and yelling at Dana that she was the meanest mom in the entire world. At the table, as Paige pouted and refused to touch her food, Dana would smile to herself, reveling in the comfort of knowing that she was a good mom who ensured her daughters' health and protected them from a toxic food system. She had neither given up nor given in. That's what Dana would have done in this parallel universe.

But that was not the universe Dana lived in. That evening, Dana was completely at the end of her rope after five days of hospital shifts and her unhappy discovery, earlier that afternoon, of a utility bill double what she had expected.

So Dana made compromises that kept her kids happy and

calm, which, in turn, allowed her to keep putting one foot in front of the other. Internally, Dana did the emotion work to feel better about the compromises. Framing her kids' diets as an aberration helped her downplay the gaps between her dietary aspirations and their dietary reality.

Dana and Lorena did the same kind of emotion work in comparing their current situations to past, more difficult, ones. Some single mothers who had been previously partnered or married noted that feeding was less stressful now. They no longer had to cook for a "deadbeat ex-husband" or a partner who'd been "a grown-ass kid." There was one fewer person to shop for, one fewer palate to cater to, and one fewer plate to clean. It was all so much easier.

But I knew that *easier* didn't necessarily mean *easy*. For Dana, domestic life may have been more peaceful without her ex-husband, Chris, but it was still incredibly tough. Like two-thirds of single moms in this country, Dana didn't receive child support from either Madison's or Paige's father. It was stressful and taxing for Dana to cover her own and her two daughters' needs on her salary alone. Dana's father helped her out with a bit of money each month, and other family members could also be tapped in a pinch. But mostly, Dana was on her own.

I sometimes wondered about the long-term effects of this pervasive stress on moms like Dana. A growing body of research shows that chronic stress is a central mechanism through which living in poverty has a negative impact on kids and adults alike. The ongoing stresses of poverty lead to a constant release of stress hormones. These stress hormones create ongoing wear and tear on the body, which can dysregulate and damage a person's physiological stress response system, reduce cognitive and psychological resources for battling adversity, and increase the risk for a range of mental and physical problems.[4] While I saw Dana tamp down her stress through downscaling, I knew that didn't mean the stress went away. It lay heavy on her chest, a constant weight that stopped her from ever fully breathing easy. Dana knew she didn't have a safety net wide enough to catch her and the girls if something went really wrong.

Dana often fantasized about leaving all the stress behind. "The Bay Area is too expensive," she said one evening as she walked me out to my car, the sound of crickets echoing all around us. "And there's too much drama."

That drama came from many sides, but I was privy to the kind emanating directly from Chris, whom I'd had the "misery of meeting"—as Dana put it—multiple times. Some nights, Chris appeared unexpectedly at Dana's front door, reeking of cigarettes and beer. Before he arrived on one Wednesday evening, after what had been one of the hottest days of summer, Dana and I were plopped side by side on the couch. Dana scrolled with an index finger through photos on her phone, showing me professional ones of her and the girls from last year at their neighborhood park. When Chris showed up, wearing his usual T-shirt and trucker hat, Dana asked him for money for back-to-school supplies. Dana hated having to ask. She wished Chris would just offer, like he was supposed to. But Dana was running short that month and needed him to pitch in. Right hand on her hip, Dana showed Chris a receipt from Target for notebooks, pencils, a ruler, and crayons.

"You think I don't believe you?" Chris joked, his defensiveness piercing the air. "I got you, home slice."

But Chris didn't have her. With each passing minute, Dana grew frustrated as Chris somehow found a way to keep skirting the issue and avoid paying up. After he drove off without committing to anything, Dana looked at me with visible exasperation.

"He's a mess." She rolled her eyes. "You see he's a mess, right? You don't have to lie."

Dana fell back onto the couch, stuffing the receipt in her front pocket. "Write down for your thing that being a single—a broken-home mom—is tough."

I wrote it down and underlined it twice.

But just a half hour later, Dana acted like it hadn't happened. "That's our life, nothing too exciting!" she said cheerily as we folded Paige's leotards and Madison's tank tops.

Dana was downscaling her frustration and exasperation to normalize everything. At times like this, I saw that downscaling wasn't just about coming to terms with reality. It was also a way of preserving dignity, of being the hero of one's own story rather than the victim. Dana had been a victim several times: of sexual assault, intimate-partner violence, cancer, and, now, two negligent fathers to her two children. But Dana didn't want to see herself that way. It was exhausting and depleting to focus on those stories. So Dana did the emotion work to spin the situation and see it in a brighter light. She took control of the narrative and came out on top.

Another evening a few weeks later, Dana opened the door to find Chris filling the door frame, a white plastic trash bag slung over his shoulder. The bag was overflowing with Paige's clothes that hadn't been washed in months. When Dana opened the bag, an unmistakable stench of smoke and alcohol filled their tiny kitchen. Dana's eyes welled up as she knelt on the white tiles and stuffed the clothes into the washing machine. I helped her, breathing through my mouth to let the stench pass. But fifteen minutes later, with the laundry running and Dana at the kitchen sink washing up from dinner, she casually commented, "Just another boring night at home."

Even when things were tough, even when Dana's tears overcame her, she continually worked to downplay it, to reframe challenging, stressful occurrences as uneventful. She did the internal work to feel that things were normal even when her raw emotions revealed that they were, in fact, not. She undertook the internal efforts to save face, not so much for me as for herself. When I once asked her if she'd ever remarry, Dana gave me a bewildered look. Why would she do that? She squinted at me. Things were perfectly great on her own.

CHAPTER 17

Upscaling

It was often the wealthiest, most privileged moms who emanated the most stress, worry, and uncertainty about their kids' diets. At first, this confused me. From where I was sitting, affluent moms had reason to feel pretty good about what their kids were eating. Were their children perfect angels who always ate all their peas and never asked for cake? No, but with all the resources these moms possessed to make feeding easier, their concerns felt disproportionate to their circumstances. Why didn't they exude an air of confidence and comfort that reflected their positions of privilege?

Wealthier moms' anxieties about getting kids' diets "right" were embedded within a much broader, deeper class anxiety that has characterized privileged parenting in the United States for at least the past thirty years. Sociologists have shown that growing economic inequality and uncertainty have augmented wealthier parents' stress about their children getting and staying ahead. These parents want their children to enjoy the same financial and educational advantages they have but see such advantages as harder to guarantee. Many parents are aware, for instance, that the competition for admission to elite colleges and universities has skyrocketed since the 1970s. Parents' fears about children's futures reflect their awareness that in an increasingly winner-takes-all society, their kids are at risk of losing.[1]

Moms saw kids' diets as key to them winning. As Latisha—the

socially mobile mom from chapter 9—knew, what kids ate could facilitate or impede their success. It could establish them as members of the upper middle class, or it could drag them into a lower social stratum. Food's consequentiality placed a burden on moms. Moms shouldered that burden and ran with it—constantly questioning their feeding strategies, second-guessing whether they were doing enough to get their kids the "best" foods, wondering whether they were cutting out enough of the "bad" stuff, and fearing they weren't successfully instilling nutritional values in their kids that would ensure their long-term health.

Instead of downscaling their feelings or putting the situation in perspective, these moms often did the exact opposite. They increased the effort and mental energy spent on feeding their children. They did this by *upscaling,* or constantly ratcheting up the standards by which they evaluated their kids' diets and themselves as moms. In their minds, they never did enough, and upscaling helped fuel such feelings of inadequacy on a daily basis. Simply put, wealthy moms dealt with their deep-seated worries about what their kids ate by worrying even more. While low-income moms' downscaling helped align expectations with reality, high-income moms' upscaling widened the gap between expectations and reality. Upscaling not only led these moms to raise their standards; it was also a tool to manage their anxieties through engendering a sense of being in control of a situation that could often feel uncontrollable.

If lower-income moms applied a wider lens to put things in perspective—comparing their current diets to what they'd eaten in earlier, more difficult times—their wealthier counterparts took a microscope to the issue, drilling in on all sorts of shortcomings and challenges. Wealthier moms were quick to identify problems with their kids' diets, including their bad habits and guilty pleasures. They were also quick to point out places where they, as moms, were failing. Self-deprecating comments were so common I started a list to keep track. Sometimes these comments were as specific and concise as Julie's admission that "usually we don't eat breakfast, which is terrible because it's the most important meal of the day." Other times, such comments permeated longer monologues about parenting failures, like one mom's confession of guilt "for not giving my children all the things that I know that they could do better with."

Moms were also resolute that they should be able to solve these problems. They should be able to break their kids' Cocoa Krispies cravings or get them to like cauliflower—and they should be doing it *now*. As moms created and fixated on these challenges, they raised the bar to a level that was incredibly high and usually unrealistic. They set themselves up to fall short.

How high was the bar moms were trying to vault? While it varied, most moms were trying to surmount the unreasonably lofty standard set by intensive mothering—the one that told them they should be child-centered, self-sacrificing, and protective in their feeding practices. Most moms bought into these tenets. They felt that they should be regularly preparing homemade meals for their kids. But above this already high bar, many moms also believed—unrealistically, from my perspective— that their kids should want, or even prefer, their cooking to fast food or takeout. Moms thought that they should be so talented at feeding that their kids would run home after school, breezing by the gas station with its shelves of candy, and beg for their moms' lasagnas, dumplings, *migas,* or biryani.

What made the high bar moms set even less achievable was that it happened to be a moving target—the closer a mom got to it, the higher it could be raised. The only thing moms could count on was that it would always be out of reach.

This was the experience of Janae Lathrop, the mother of three I introduced in chapter 10. As Janae and I drank our fruit smoothies in her brightly lit living room, she told me about her experiences trying to integrate the fresh food she loved with the soul food she'd grown up with. But time was not on Janae's side. Monday through Friday, Janae took the train into San Francisco for work and then back home, an hour each way. With her two-hour daily commute and her responsibility for feeding the family, Janae was often stretched thin and stressed out. She felt like she wasn't measuring up. Janae wanted her daughters to eat healthy, but couldn't always make that happen.

Mostly, she said, "It's the dinner thing that we have to figure out." Dinner had been a struggle for years. Last year, Janae's long work hours brought her to the point where they were eating takeout most evenings. Even now, she guiltily told me, she resorted to takeout at least once a week. "Currently I'm still probably doing—I want to say one day a week pickup. There was a point in time where we did, like, three days a week. People, they all know me. Like, I would just call, and they would say, 'Hi, Janae! Your usual? Yeah, okay. Bye-bye!' And they would meet me on the road." Janae set her glass down on the table. "It's embarrassing."

Things came to a head for Janae when her daughters divulged to their grandmother—Janae's mother—that Janae was feeding them Chinese food and pizza most nights.

"One time, my mom asked my children, 'What does Mommy cook for you each night?' And they said, 'Whatever's in the bag,' meaning the takeout bag. And I was crushed. As a mom, talk about guilt. I'm like, 'Oh my goodness.' I didn't have that experience. My mom never bought takeout. Her food was better than the takeout." Janae shook her head ruefully, tucking the wisps of black hair around her face back into her bun. For Janae, relying on takeout was akin to failing. It was also humiliating. "Can I not figure this out?" Janae had asked herself. "To be a mom— a working mom?"

If Janae's idea of figuring it out involved zero takeout and all homemade meals, then from my perspective, the answer to her question was likely no. These were tall orders that would probably demand that Janae stay at home rather than work full-time. So far, I'd seen only moms like Julie pull that off—and even they still felt guilty about perceived shortcomings! For years, women, and mothers in particular, have been repeatedly told that it's possible to "have it all"—to raise a family, work full-time, keep up hobbies, and feel a sense of balance. Moms like Janae wanted this to be true. They worked hard to make this true. But this wasn't true because society has never been set up to make it true. In the United States, unrealistically high expectations for moms' obligations to their families have been accompanied by a glaring absence of structural supports—things like paid leave and flexible work hours—to meet those expectations.

But Janae was more optimistic than me. She decided that she could have it all—but only by getting a new job. When I met Janae, she had been in her new role for four months. While the hours were still long, they were more manageable. Janae now had time to prepare weeknight dinners. But Janae's honeymoon period after the job change was short-lived. She quickly found new ways to raise the bar for herself and, in doing so, convince herself that she was still disappointing. Janae was now making dinners regularly during the week, but she started to feel guilty that her dinners were more "semi-homemade" than "home-made." The precut vegetables and whole roasted chickens she purchased became a new source of embarrassment. Was she giving it her all if dinner took only a few minutes to come together?

Janae's original goal had been to prepare more dinners at home. But that goal soon vanished, replaced by a new one. Now "homemade" meant "from scratch." It meant using raw, whole ingredients. It meant lots of prep work—cutting, chopping, peeling—and, ideally, at least an hour of cooking time. It meant using a recipe. Unless dinner was a hot meal that Janae had planned out and over which she had labored for hours, she felt that what she was offering her daughters just wasn't good enough.

"Trader Joe's even has the whole thing that you toss with the sauce," Janae told me, referring to a salad kit that came with its own dressing. She rolled her eyes. "I'm like, 'You're kidding!' It's almost embarrassing because I think literally, one time, dinner was done in five minutes. Like, the chicken lasagna. Here's a salad. Everyone's happy. Everyone's happy."

Gesturing toward the kitchen where the frozen chicken lasagna was presumably waiting, Janae sighed. "It's like we're cheating."

As our conversation continued, Janae became increasingly convinced that she was going to make some big changes to her family's diet. Meeting me, she said, grinning, was motivating her. Indeed, my mere presence seemed to amplify moms' desires to upscale. Our conversations brought moms' feelings of guilt to the surface and intensified their desire to alleviate those feelings through action. Some interviews ended with moms compiling a laundry list of dietary improvements they were going to implement once I left.

"So I'm actually at that place where this is important for me to do." Janae leaned forward, clasping her hands. "I mean, literally even beyond this study I was actually like, 'Okay. How can I do this? How can I do this?'" Janae was determined to have it all—to thrive professionally and win at intensive mothering. She could work nine to five *and* give her kids healthy, home-made food. Minutes later, Janae jumped up from the couch to retrieve three cookbooks from the bookshelf. She came back, and together, we flipped through the pages of Chrissy Teigen's *Cravings,* which featured recipes like spicy tomato skillet eggs, vegetable tortilla soup, and a "dump and done" ramen salad. We discussed which dishes Janae could try that week, and she started jotting down the ingredients for a sesame chicken noodle dish.

When Janae said our conversation motivated her, it was like she thought I was actively encouraging her to make changes. In reality, I had posed non-leading, open-ended questions, nodded along, and taken notes. I had assured her that I was a sociologist, not a nutritionist or a pediatrician interested in evaluating anything. But simply talking about how their kids ate unearthed moms' deep-seated feelings of inadequacy. Once those feelings were on the table, moms like Janae felt they had no choice but to raise the bar once again. They wanted me to know that they were committed to doing better, and there was no amount of reassurance I could offer to stop moms from judging themselves. While lower-income moms navigated that judgment by trying to make everything feel okay, wealthier moms navigated it by demonstrating that they were committed to doing a better job.

It wasn't just working moms like Janae who struggled with their own ever-rising standards. Even stay-at-home parents who were already regularly preparing home-cooked meals from scratch felt that there was significant room for improvement.

Joaquin Vargas was one such parent. Joaquin, a short, lean man with kind eyes and a receding hairline, was the only stay-at-home father I interviewed. He was also an anomaly in the United States, where only 7 percent of fathers are full-time caregivers to their children (compared to 27 percent of mothers).[2] A dad of two, he was also one of four dads in my study of seventy-five families who was primarily in charge of food.

"Growing up, we ate whatever was available," Joaquin told me about his childhood diet in Bolivia. "A lot of starch, rice, potato, a lot of meat. A lot of soda. It was never questioned. Sugar everywhere. MSG, it was actually part of every meal."

When Joaquin moved to the States and met his nutrition-oriented wife in graduate school, everything changed. After quitting his job to become a stay-at-home father, he was determined to raise his son and daughter on a diet that was healthy, unprocessed, and free of pesticides and chemicals. To achieve this, Joaquin prepared their food from scratch, using a combination of the vegetables he grew in his backyard garden and organic produce from the farmers' markets. When I interviewed his kids, fourteen-year-old Xavier and twelve-year-old Ellie, in their bright, minimalist house one afternoon, I found Joaquin in the kitchen rolling out the crust for a quiche and chopping vegetables for a salad.

Joaquin didn't just cook food. He talked constantly to his children about it. "I tell them about how I was raised and how wrong it was," Joaquin said, slicing an orange pepper. "How nobody questioned it. How having means is good. Why it's important for them to study so they can buy better food and so they can buy a big lot so they can grow vegetables in the back, or fruit trees. So I don't push things on them, but I tell them constantly."

Xavier and Ellie confirmed that their dad talked to them incessantly about food. " 'Vegetables! Eat vegetables! And milk's good. It helps your bones grow. And sugar is poison!' " Ellie laughed, imitating her dad.

While Joaquin felt that he was feeding his children better than he had been fed as a child, he was also in a state of worry that his efforts were falling short. And he made sure his children knew this, because he never wanted them to settle for anything less than the best.

"Now they know that stir-fry is good but not that good, that I'm trying to figure out ways to make it better," he explained. "We have to work on that in the near future."

When it came to his kids' diets, Joaquin was an optimizer. Each day, Joaquin learned more and more about what foods and means of preparation were healthiest, continually refining his approach as his knowledge deepened. He read newspapers, perused blogs, and stayed up-to-date on the latest nutrition studies. When nutrition experts' opinions changed, so did Joaquin's. Recently, Joaquin had discovered that reduced-fat milk was healthier than the nonfat milk his family had been drinking. The next day, Joaquin switched out the kids' dairy. Xavier and Ellie didn't like the taste of the new milk at first, but Joaquin stuck to his guns. "They had a hard time adjusting." He smiled. "But they did over two weeks or three weeks."

Joaquin wasn't alone on his endless quest for nutritional information and improvement; he turned to the media, friends, and fellow parents for dietary advice. But this relentless digestion of information seemed only to intensify his anxieties that he wasn't doing enough. Despite Joaquin's staggering efforts to keep up — to find and feed his kids the "ideal diet" — he was still plagued by a gnawing sense of inadequacy. "I think I'm doing fine but I'm not doing great," he confessed. "I want to do great."

When I asked Joaquin what he meant by that, he explained that he wanted more information and clear guidance. "I wish someone would say, 'This is the right thing to do.' There isn't. Like right now, at forty-eight years old, I don't know how much better it is to steam broccoli instead of roasting it for a few minutes. People tell me no, it's good fresh. Is that necessarily the truth?" Joaquin sighed. "I don't know."

I couldn't help thinking that perhaps it wasn't an accident that Joaquin didn't know — that perhaps the goal of media outlets, health blogs, and the food industry was to keep people guessing. Or, setting my cynicism aside, at the very least they probably weren't trying to clear up the confusion. Dissent — not consensus — sells. The media always need new nutrition stories to print, and health bloggers depend on making strong claims to draw viewers repeatedly to sites. The food industry profits from keeping people confused so that they continue buying its spurious health claims and its products.

I could see how this confusion played out in my own nutritional knowledge over time. It seemed like certain foods' popularity and supposed healthiness vacillated widely every few years, going from healthy to unhealthy, from good to bad. For years, we knew that butter was terrible for us...until it wasn't. Sugar was supposedly fine for consumption...until it wasn't. Fad diets' promise and popularity were just as fleeting. I distinctly remember when the Atkins, Paleo, keto, and Mediterranean diets debuted, each supposedly offering the solution to our nation's dietary woes. Rather than a surprise, Joaquin's confusion seemed like the natural consequence of this persistent, pervasive, and puzzling nutritional discourse. And in upscaling, he and other high-income parents found a way to channel the anxiety about that uncertainty into action.

As much time as Joaquin spent reading blogs and scanning media outlets, he lamented that he didn't "have the time to research every little thing." And like Janae, talking with me only upped Joaquin's motivation to institute changes he'd been toying with. Rolling up the sleeves of his North Face fleece, Joaquin said, "Having this conversation with you is making me reflect more on what I'm doing. It's like talking to a psychologist because you do all the talking and then you're like, 'Huh, that's right, I can change this!'"

CHAPTER 18

Priorities

"What keeps you up at night?" I asked Lorena Garcia in the living room of the thirteen-hundred-square-foot apartment she rented for her boyfriend, daughter, son, and two grandchildren.

Lorena stared at me, stone-faced. Every night when her cheek hit the pillow, the same fear flashed before her eyes. "I worry that I'm going to wake up to the police knocking on my door, telling me my son's been shot," she said, looking down at her feet.

Three months earlier, Lorena's son Alejandro had been recruited into a gang. He was nineteen years old with a son of his own and a steady girlfriend, and Lorena had hoped that Alejandro's new family responsibilities would keep him on the straight and narrow. "You have people who depend on you now," she'd told him a year ago when he moved out of her house and into an apartment with his girlfriend and son. But Alejandro had gotten caught up in the wrong crowd, and now Lorena didn't know where he went most evenings. He didn't have a job, and his girlfriend cared for their child. Lorena felt frustrated, but that frustration was overshadowed by her fears of the worst possible outcome. If it happened, she said with a sigh, Alejandro wouldn't be the first person she'd loved to die by gunshot.

In the face of the very real possibility of losing her son, Lorena rearranged her priorities. Food wasn't at the top of the list. Her most pressing concern wasn't whether she was getting Alejandro to eat enough broccoli or whether she could help curb her younger daughter's chip cravings. Lorena was not alone; many lower-income moms worried about things that never crossed affluent moms' radars. Some feared for their children's safety walking to and from school. Others worried about their kids' security once they were home, alone, waiting for an adult to return from work. Others were seriously concerned about their children not completing school at all. And still others feared the impacts of addiction or intimate-partner violence on their children. This is not to say that every lower-income mom worried about *all* these things. And a few didn't worry about any of them. But when these concerns came up, it was largely in conversation with lower-income moms.[1]

Kids' dietary health wasn't always the highest concern to these moms. The circumstances kids were growing up in could force low-income moms to feel just as, if not more, concerned about their kids' emotional health as their nutritional intake. For these moms, children's safety and psychological well-being—two things moms could rarely take for granted—often took precedence over healthy meals. When evictions forced families to move, when neighborhood shootings took friends' lives, when unexpected layoffs precluded medical care, or when the kitchen cupboards were empty, moms worried not about the specifics of what their kids were eating but about whether their kids were getting by—whether they were doing *okay*. Doing okay had far less to do with vegetable consumption and far more to do with staying safe and relatively happy. Doing okay meant they were staying out of the police's sight and off the school principal's suspension list.

Nyah told me that what made her happiest was knowing her girls were safe and out of harm's way. "When I hear that front door open and I know they're both in the house, I'm relieved." She smiled. "*That* brings me joy."

I realized that affluent moms were able to upscale about their kids' diets because of all the other things these moms *didn't* have to worry about. They didn't have to worry about their kids' safety, shelter, or satiety. Privileged moms could take these basic needs for granted, which freed up mental energy and space to be concerned about other aspects of their children's well-being, like their diets.

Because lower-income moms' circumstances often demanded prioritizing their kids' safety and security above all else, I saw that shifting their focus *away* from food could actually be help-ful. When the deck felt too stacked against their children eating healthy, moms focused on other aspects of their child-rearing or kids' well-being to feel like they were doing a good job. Being a good mom became less about pushing spinach and more about being present and involved in children's lives. The latter was how low-income moms enacted intensive mothering given the con-straints they faced. It was how they acted child-centered, self-sacrificing, and protective of their children. And it was how they, personally, evaluated their worth as moms.

On top of that, low-income moms were also keenly aware that opportunities to substantially improve their families' circum-stances were limited. While many hoped for a better financial future, most knew that the odds were that they would always hover at or below the poverty line. So instead of battling endlessly to bet-ter an unimprovable situation, they fought to feel better about how things were, to accept their current realities rather than constantly wish for better ones. They taught themselves to see the virtues of their kids' diets rather than the shortcomings. They focused on appreciating the food they did have rather than pining for the food they didn't. On the broadest level, they worked to feel grate-ful for what was going well and not think about what wasn't.

Dana, for instance, constantly highlighted the pride she felt about being there for Madison and Paige. While Dana wanted her daughters to eat a nutritious diet, she was generally more ori-ented toward other dimensions of their well-being that she could ensure by spending time with them and making positive memo-ries together. Having put them through a rough divorce and two moves—including a major downsizing—earlier that year, Dana was vigilant about making sure that Madison and Paige were still doing okay. She spent the limited time and money she had to throw her kids the birthday parties they wanted, get them passes to a local water park, and take them on the occasional vacation. She focused less on preparing wholesome meals and more on providing them with opportunities to get an emotional boost: a surprise trip down to Disneyland, a visit to the nail salon, a trip to Goodwill with friends.

Dana sometimes framed being there for her children as a trade-off with healthy eating. So that she could be there as much as possible for her kids, she often had to take them out to eat where they wanted and sacrifice cooking the meals she thought would be best. One evening, Madison offered to prepare a special dinner for her mom and sister. Dana, wanting to encourage Madison's independence, left the decision about what to cook up to her daughter. Dana hoped that Madison might prepare something vegetarian, but Madison told her she was going to make angel-hair pasta with beef sauce and breadsticks. Dana didn't want to upset Madison by suggesting something else or offering a critique. She knew suggesting that Madison make green beans instead of the beef would go over like a lead balloon. Dana wanted the dinner to be fun and pleasant, something that enhanced her daughter's self-esteem.

Later that evening, Dana was glad she'd bit her tongue. As Madison set the table with three black plates and three stemless glasses, the young girl's pride was as palpable as the aroma of tomato sauce filling the tiny kitchen. Madison placed a carafe of tap water in the center of the table and served each of her dining partners, beaming, as she discussed the evening's menu. As the four of us sat chatting around the table, Dana also seemed happy. "My girls love eating dinner together because they think it's so cool." She smiled, twirling the thin strands of pasta around her fork.

Another evening, as Dana leaned over the kitchen table

covered in school papers, she explained to me how her girls' childhoods diverged from her own. "Growing up, we weren't busy." She shook her head. "But me"—she paused—"I am *with* my children."

Dana had ample evidence of her involved parenting. She had countless iPhone photos of recent excursions with Madison and Paige, like a trip to the bowling alley, a Friday evening spent dyeing their hair, and a Friday afternoon spent getting their nails done at a nearby strip-mall salon. Dana's involvement in her daughters' lives was in part motivated by a deep-seated desire to keep Paige and Madison happy. Some of the involvement, though, had to do with keeping them safe. Dana worried about her daughters' safety around their neighborhood. The thought of the two of them out and about after dark on the street sent her heart racing. Theirs was a vibrant, diverse neighborhood but also one where break-ins, burglaries, and even the occasional shooting were not unheard of. Dana constantly reminded me to lock my car, and she always accompanied me to it after dark.

Safety was such a priority that Dana often spent her Friday evenings chauffeuring the girls here and there just to keep Madison from hanging out in the park with what Dana called "troublemakers." One such evening, we drove eighty minutes to get the girls bubble tea with their friends. Another afternoon, we visited Savers, a secondhand shop, where Dana let the girls try on outfits, ultimately buying them a couple of leotards, tank tops, and dresses for just over thirty dollars. Afterward, Dana told me that she had all of Madison's social media account names and passwords so that she could monitor them. "I'm involved," she said proudly.

Other moms echoed Dana's safety priorities. Ximena Gomez, a soft-spoken mom with olive skin and a wide smile, grew up in El Salvador but came to the United States with her ex-husband in the early 2000s. Living undocumented, Ximena told me, made everything more complicated. A few months before I met her, three of her five sons had been beaten up by a local gang three blocks from her house, which she shared with them and her eldest son's children. To keep her sons and their families safe, Ximena had to find a new place in a different neighborhood. But securing a new home was not easy; the housing market offered few affordable options that could fit her family. This had forced her to temporarily split the family up. She and her youngest son, Juan, lived in her car. Her older sons and their families lived with friends.

"I lost my house," Ximena told me. "They beat up Miguel and Mario, those *cholos*. Then they beat up my son Juan, and they tried to kill him. I needed to evacuate, to leave and live on the street with my children."

Other unhoused mothers told similar stories. Some of these moms lived in their cars; others with friends, family, or even coworkers. Shelters weren't good long-term options. And without documentation, Ximena couldn't apply for public housing. On the private rental market, she couldn't afford much. Even the one-bedroom she'd been renting cost her two-thirds of the income she brought in cleaning houses for thirteen dollars an hour.

Ximena felt the deep, penetrating stress of making ends meet, of keeping her kids and her grandkids clothed and fed. "It's ugly, undergoing this situation, and I wouldn't wish it on anyone," she told me. "I've lived it. There are times I don't have money for gas. I don't have any money sometimes. Life in the United States is hard if you weren't born here."

While unhoused, Ximena could not feed her youngest son, Juan, the way she wanted. "We eat in the street. We live in the street," she explained. Living in the street meant not having a kitchen to cook in or a fridge to store food. Eating in the street meant that she and Juan ate out almost every evening, mostly at fast-food chains like Pizza Hut and Kentucky Fried Chicken. Doing so not only helped stave off hunger but also offered a toilet to use and a sink to wash up in. It offered a place to sit down that wasn't Ximena's driver's seat. It offered a fleeting feeling of normalcy. When Ximena sat across from her son in a slick red booth, enough food between them to fill their stomachs, she could almost forget that they'd be retiring later that evening to lumpy, polyester seat cushions, not comforter-lined beds.

It wasn't that Ximena particularly loved fast food or thought it was a healthy choice for Juan. To the contrary, she was deeply worried about Juan's diet. "In the name of Jesus, this needs to end," she told me, running her hand through her wavy brown hair. "I need to find a place for us to live so I can make them food. Because meals are very important. The food you eat is what your body depends on, and it may help your body function. And the most important thing is having fresh food—eating healthy."

Ximena missed many things about her old house. She missed chasing her two-year-old granddaughter around its grassy backyard. She missed taking hot showers in the morning before everyone else got up. She missed evenings sprawled on the couch, sandwiched between her children, their eyes all glued to the twenty-five-inch-screen TV she'd bought them four Christmases ago. But these days, Ximena couldn't stop dreaming of her kitchen. It had been a narrow room with limited counter space and a fridge door that never reliably shut. It hadn't been perfect. But Ximena had never asked for perfect. She didn't need perfect to make her boys the squash soup she'd grown up with.

As Ximena bemoaned the reality that cooking them homemade food probably wouldn't happen for the next few weeks, if not months, I started to feel something on a uniquely emotional level. I felt a visceral anger boil up inside of me, a reaction to society's portrayals of low-income moms as too negligent or unaware to offer their kids nutritious food. Ximena's story was evidence of the level of inaccuracy, unfairness, and ignorance informing that portrayal.

Ximena was neither negligent nor unaware. She knew the

trade-offs she was making. She'd done the calculations. In the end, she had chosen—as any parent in her situation would—to prioritize Juan's life over his diet. Ximena had stared down the constellation of impossibly difficult circumstances facing her and her family and made the necessary sacrifices to overcome them. Right now, Ximena decided, her kids' lives were simply more important than their fruit and vegetable consumption.

Ximena did her best with that difficult hand she had been dealt. Even though she and her kids were without a home, she focused on the few ways that she was still able to do right by them. She worried less about controlling their diets and more about how she could meet their emotional needs—their desire to feel loved and cared for by their mom, to feel "normal."

"They say, 'I want McDonald's. I want Taco Bell. I want Pollo Loco. I want Carl's Junior. I want Chinese food.'" Ximena rolled her eyes. With limited opportunities to meet their needs elsewhere, Ximena told me, she generally tried to oblige. She tried to take them each to their favorite place at least once a week.

"In other words," Ximena said with a grin, "I give everyone the same privilege, always everyone. So that they're happy. For me, all of them are equal. Because all of them are my children, and I adore all of them very much, and I want the best for them."

Ximena did not feel great about her family's current diet, but she worked hard on her emotions to create a feeling of comfort—calm, even—in the midst of a heart-wrenching situation. She fought to downplay her struggles and frustrations so as not to be reduced by the current tumult. She assured herself that good moms always found a way to make sure their kids came out on top. Ximena had done it before, and she would do it again. When she sacrificed to keep her kids safe and when she treated each of them equally and with respect, she did right by them. By concentrating on these positives, Ximena leveraged an awe-inspiring emotional resourcefulness, restoring her sense of dignity in a context meant to strip her of it.

CHAPTER 19

Control

While low-income moms' extremely challenging circumstances could force a de-prioritization of their kids' diets, the opposite was true for wealthier moms: their privileged contexts seemed to fuel a hyper-prioritization of kids' consumption. While low-income moms downscaled to worry less about controlling their kids' diets, high-income moms upscaled—fretting about and fighting to control what went into their kids' bodies.

In just a few months, Patricia Adams's eldest daughter, Zoe, would be heading off to college. Patricia, whom we met in chapter 8, would miss Zoe. After eighteen years under Patricia's watch, Zoe would be on her own soon, an independent young adult solely responsible for her three daily meals, not to mention snacks, drinks, and desserts.

But as long as Zoe was still under this roof, Patricia said with a laugh, she was subject to her mom's dietary rules and meddling. As long as Patricia continued to buy Zoe's food and make Zoe's meals, Zoe's consumption was still very much Patricia's business.

"I still try to control her!" Patricia chuckled. "I'm still going, 'You need to eat five bites of zucchini! You need your vitamins!'"

Zoe's diet mattered to Patricia because its impacts were far-reaching. Eating zucchini today wasn't important solely because it boosted Zoe's current vitamin C intake; those bites of green portended her future vegetable consumption. If Zoe binged on Skittles now, the stomachache that would quickly follow wasn't the only problem; too much sugar in this moment could drive Zoe's sugar addiction later. Zoe's present food choices would shape her future diet and health, and Patricia wanted to ensure that future was as bright as possible.

As I explained in chapter 17, privileged moms' anxieties about their kids' welfare are embedded within an overarching, gnawing class anxiety that characterizes modern parenthood. Parents' deep-seated fears that their children might descend a few rungs on the socioeconomic ladder, losing whatever class advantages they currently possess, has motivated what the economists Garey and Valerie Ramey call the "rug rat race."[1] In this race, parents direct more and more resources to parenting and kids' enrichment activities. Indeed, compared to earlier generations of caregivers, parents today devote significantly more time and attention to their children. Wealthier parents also spend more money on kids than they used to—and more than other American families can currently afford to. Affluent parents hope that, together, their temporal, cognitive, and monetary investments will land their kids spots at elite universities and secure them well-paying jobs. But there also exists a gulf between affluent parents' hopes for their kids and the limits of parents' power to achieve those hopes. This gulf can be extremely anxiety-provoking, as parents have to confront wanting something so badly for their kids but also being unable to guarantee it. How do parents navigate this frustrating reality?

One answer is control. Wealthy parents can try to control as much as possible to increase their chances of attaining the desired outcome. Over the years, catchy terms have popped up to capture these controlling trends in parenting. *Helicopter parenting*, for instance, refers to parental overinvolvement and overregulation of kids' lives. Helicopter parents, so named because they "hover overhead" like helicopters, take a risk-averse approach to child-rearing, overseeing every aspect of their kids' lives and working to protect them from outside risks and harm. The more recent term *snowplow parenting* describes parents who go one step further, trying, like a snowplow, to preemptively remove any obstacles that might delay or prevent their kids' success.[2]

While parents across society work to control aspects of children's lives, wealthier parents take a heavier-handed approach, as the sociologist Annette Lareau discovered through her research of parenting practices in the 1990s. Through interviews and observations of families, Lareau found that more privileged parents raised kids differently than lower-income families and that these differences cut across racial lines. The former engaged in what she called *concerted cultivation*—they viewed parenting as a highly hands-on, labor-intensive project meant to provide children with skills, activities, and behaviors that would secure future privileges. Lareau contrasted this approach with a less-hands-on parenting style she called *the accomplishment of natural growth* that was more common among lower-income parents.[3]

The affluent parents I met practiced the concerted cultivation that Lareau wrote about twenty years ago. But the same anxieties that drove those parents to practice concerted cultivation also led them to engage in what I came to see as the *physical cultivation* of their children. When parents worked to physically cultivate their kids, they did so by instilling in kids the knowledge, habits, and beliefs about food and health they hoped would grant them advantages later on.

Patricia was painfully aware of all that she couldn't control. She couldn't know what her younger two daughters would score on their SATs or whether they'd earn spots on the varsity volleyball team. But their diets were something different.

"What you eat, it's something that you can control," she said, a grin sweeping across her face. "There are so many factors that collide that you have no control over. For me, if I can control our food, it's one less thing that's in that equation."

Some moms were not comfortable discussing control as

overtly as Patricia. Many couched their efforts to control in softer language, telling me that they focused on "guiding smart choices" and "offering good options." When I asked moms if they had any rules at home around food, some quickly delivered a hard no before then sharing a list of "guidelines," "habits," or "best practices" they generally stuck to. Certainly, some affluent moms took a more free-range approach to their kids' diets, highlighting the importance of moderation and accepting junk and fast food as a natural, pleasant part of childhood. These moms felt great pride in their comparatively laissez-faire approach, which highlighted the double standards of lower- and higher-income parenting. When lower-income moms were less hands-on with their kids' diets, they were generally labeled negligent or ignorant. When wealthier moms practiced the same thing, they were perceived as less overbearing and applauded for fostering their kids' independence and creativity. The same parenting practices did not garner the same societal evaluations.

Yet even the less controlling affluent moms knew that they *could* intervene and exert control if necessary. How did they know this? One reason, I learned, was that wealthier moms (and the majority were white) were simply accustomed to having more control when it came to child-rearing. In general, these moms could afford to live where they wanted, send their kids to their preferred schools, secure the best tutors, and enroll their kids in the extracurricular activities of their choice. What went into their kids' bodies was like any other aspect of kids' lives that moms oversaw and managed. What's more, not having the worries that kept low-income moms up at night, high-income moms dug their heels into that management. They were poised to jump in and fix any problems that arose. And problems in need of fixing, I learned, arose often.

For Patricia, opportunities for physical cultivation were abundant and helped her feel like she had some authority over her kids even as they grew up. Food was as omnipresent as opportunities to regulate it. Moms helped kids pick their science classes once a year, but they could guide their food choices anywhere from three to thirteen times a day. Kids were constantly making dietary decisions, whether it was what to eat for breakfast, what snacks to pack for soccer practice, where to eat with their friends after school, or how many helpings to take for dinner. Patricia had endless chances to insert "teaching moments," to make humble suggestions to eat this and not that, and to put together a plate with just the right balance of food groups.

Children's diets and bodies were also highly visible to moms. If ignorance is bliss, then for moms, seeing everything their kids ate was hell. Moms noticed when the box of Milanos in the cupboard emptied more quickly than usual or when kids put on weight. Moms monitored their kids' dietary intake by tracking which foods disappeared and when. Food's visibility only dialed up moms' attention and stress levels. With their kids' "poor" choices or missteps constantly on display, moms felt the urgency of course-correcting before it grew too late—before one bag of M&M's turned into two, or twelve.

Moms' physical cultivation of kids began early and stemmed from simply following prescriptive guidelines. As society's shepherds of children's health, mothers in the United States are trained early and repeatedly to feel that deep, personal sense of ownership over their kids' intake. This responsibility for physically cultivating children begins in pregnancy with directions to take prenatal vitamins and avoid coffee and cold cuts. It continues into the newborn phase with the public health guidance to exclusively breastfeed babies for at least six months. It carries into infancy with advice for the best ways to expose a child to solid foods and into toddlerdom and childhood with the clear advice to avoid sugar-sweetened products. Through it all, kids' weights are fastidiously monitored in pediatricians' offices, with slight deviations in weight, height, or BMI percentiles flagged as evidence of something wrong—of a failure on the part of moms. My daughter's weight had received a grade during her first visit to the pediatrician, and other moms are subject to their own scores. From the time of baby bumps onward, moms get the clear message that being a good mother means controlling their kids' intake and bodies.

Privileged moms with resources are positioned to act on that message. Many such moms told me that their earliest, sharpest memories had to do with feeding their infants. Many followed the "breast is best" approach. As Janae Lathrop said, "I was that anal mom with children. They never had a jar of baby food. And I was all about, 'Oh, let me cook my own applesauce and smash my own bananas.' And why buy bananas baby food? You can do your own." This philosophy of responsibility and control evolved as kids grew. For the moms I met, years of nursing and pureeing sweet potatoes gave way to sugar-free birthday cakes and packed lunches. It fueled efforts to keep kids away from juice and soda and expose them to a range of fruits and vegetables. All of it was hard, but the teenage years were when things started to get even trickier. Controlling a five-year-old's diet was a bit easier than regulating a fourteen-year-old's. With their increasing autonomy, independent spending power, and outside social lives, teens made moms feel that they were losing their grip. Physical cultivation grew even more challenging.

Moms' fears of dissipating influence only fueled their anxiety. To navigate it, they searched tirelessly for ways—big and small— to exercise control over their teens' diets. They sought avenues to slip in fruits over candy, to substitute baked chips for Ding Dongs, to swap lettuce wraps for burger buns. Moms knew that their supervision had its limits and that when teens joined their friends at the movies or biked downtown after school, they ate and drank whatever they wanted. Moms understood their reach could extend only so far. But as long as moms were constantly striving to improve their kids' consumption, then, at the very least, they could go to bed at night feeling like they were mothering well. Whatever the outcomes, no one could say they hadn't tried.

Ironically, trying to control their kids often heightened moms' worries. When their efforts failed, it left them feeling frustrated and inadequate. Because moms saw their kids' diets as controllable, they interpreted any inability to control them as a personal failure.

Weight was a key metric that moms used to deem their feeding efforts a success or a failure. A teenager's weight was measurable and visible. It was the physical manifestation of what kids were consuming—the evidence of whether moms had done a good or bad job. And it was also tracked by doctors and schools, meaning that moms were constantly grading and being graded on the numbers that appeared on the scale.

Almost every mom thought about their kids' weight, although how they did so differed. Among higher-income families, often white or Asian, moms talked more about the importance of being thin. This was especially the case when it came to their daughters. Some encouraged their daughters to watch their weight because, as one mom put it, "Once you gain it, it's hard to lose." Some moms framed a desire for their daughters' thinness as wanting better for their daughters than they had, referring to their own struggles to lose or manage their weight. This premium on thinness also applied to sons, although there was much more leeway; moms were inclined to accept their sons' heavier bodies as "athletic," sturdy, or husky.

Black and Latina mothers generally held a more inclusive image of an appropriate body size. Their daughters needn't necessarily be thin so much as "healthy." Curves were good. Being too thin was worse than being a little heavy.

Many high-income moms were also wary of compounding kids'—most often, daughters'—body-image issues or fueling eating disorders by emphasizing weight too much. They were careful not to overtly discuss weight with their kids even as they engaged in an internal dialogue about it. This put moms in a difficult position—they cared deeply about how much their kid weighed but couldn't speak openly with them about it. So instead, moms tried to control kids' diets in ways that would produce thinness, or at least a pediatrician-approved BMI. Rather than discussing pounds and ounces, they strove to get their kids to focus on being "healthy" and "feeling good."

Moms whose kids' weight deviated from the normal BMI range often tried to rein that weight in themselves. Others turned to more interventionist methods. Julie and Zach, for instance, had hired a nutritionist and a therapist a year earlier to help Jane bring her weight down. "When you see someone that you love who has a belly and who eats a cupcake and immediately after can eat again," Julie said, "it can be disturbing and not in the best interest of that person." Julie hoped Jane would learn how to exercise self-control and make "better" choices around food. But after watching Jane get bullied at school for being chubby, Julie also just wanted to help restore her daughter's confidence. Julie wanted Jane to fit in, make friends, and feel good about her appearance. If losing some weight could help achieve that, then Julie would help her daughter slim down.

The nutritionist had introduced the Cains to a system akin to Weight Watchers, complete with a hierarchy of green, yellow, and red foods to guide daily choices. "Green foods are foods that you can eat all the time that include your fruits and your vegetables and your lean proteins and your complex carbohydrates," Julie explained. Yellow foods were other meats, nuts, cheeses, and dairy. And then you had red foods. "French fries are a red food!" she said, laughing and taking a sip of carbonated water.

Julie tried to go by the nutritionist's guidelines when she grocery shopped. She bought more green foods and fewer red foods. But she genuinely worried when she saw Jane bake a batch of cookies and scarf down one after the other without pause. Julie explained to me, with a heavy sigh, that she could only give her kids information and it was their choice what they did with it. But I could tell that taking on a purely information-giving role could feel too hands-off for her. It stressed Julie out to leave Jane to her own devices. So Julie was constantly finding small ways to micromanage and steer the situation, whether it was asking Jane whether she was still hungry after her third cookie or piling the shopping cart to the brim with fruits so Jane would *want* to make the healthy choice herself. When Jane went to Starbucks with her friends, Julie reminded her daughter that she could amend her usual Frappuccino order to err on the healthier side: "Get the fat-free Frappuccino instead of the full-fat Frappuccino," Julie advised. "It'll save you so much in calories."

Virginia Bowen, a stay-at-home mom of two, found herself in a similar position. The two moms knew each other: Julie had hired Virginia's youngest son, Liam, to tutor Jane in math. Virginia was deeply committed to her sons' diets, which meant that she often felt tormented by them. I first met Virginia one morning at her home. With her black Lululemon leggings, a bright blue Nike tank top, and chestnut brown hair pulled back into a messy, sporty bun, Virginia looked like the personal trainer she worked part-time as. Virginia's world revolved around healthy eating. As her husband told me, her space was "nutrition and fitness and health and everything."

Virginia was avid about her two sons' physical cultivation and tried to keep a tight grip on what they ate. Recently, though, she'd felt that grip loosening as her sons grew from scraggly kids who liked to run around the yard to teenagers who were more interested in staring at their phones and playing video games with their friends. As Virginia and I sat down to chat at her oak dining table, she blurted out that her older son, Wells, was overweight.

Virginia was frustrated, embarrassed, and shocked that after a lifetime of trying to instill in him an appreciation for healthy food, Wells didn't care one bit about his weight or his health. For the past sixteen years, she'd tried to model a healthy diet for him. "I do not understand how I can do that," she lamented, "and I have a kid who overeats."

Wells's current diet worried Virginia in more ways than she could count. For one, she didn't like the idea of her pediatrician or other moms judging her because of how her son looked. It was embarrassing, she admitted, for a fitness instructor to have an overweight son who didn't care about any of the healthy habits so core to her whole existence. But she also worried about Wells's future, fearing the way the habits he picked up today would affect how he fared tomorrow. Watching his current poor eating choices and his reluctance to adhere to even one bullet point of her advice only entrenched Virginia's feeling of dread about whether his tastes would ever improve. Would Wells one day see the light?

"From a psychology point of view," she said, "I super-worry about his weight. I feel like I sort of lost that battle. It's one of my greatest angsts in life." Despite feeling like she was failing, Virginia never gave up trying to set a good example. When I asked her whether she thought that approach was working, she replied, dejectedly, "Ask me in ten years. I think modeling good food behavior is really important, but I don't know yet because I'm not seeing the effect."

Some of Virginia's anxiety stemmed from this frustrating truth: She was doing everything she could to fix Wells's diet, but nothing seemed to be working. Wells's hoarding and bingeing habits were starting to take on a life of their own, and that felt unfamiliar to Virginia. As a mom, Virginia was accustomed to having a handle on her family and her kids. Experiencing her control erode was confusing and upsetting.

But failure only made Virginia upscale more fervently and strive even harder to fix the problem. She reevaluated and re-strategized. She tried talking to Wells. She tried listening. She tried bribing. She even gave praying a shot. Recently, she had transitioned from trying to persuade Wells to eat healthy to just giving him and his younger brother what she thought they should be eating. On her kitchen counter that afternoon I spotted a bowl of grapes and a plate of baby carrots. "I pretty much just put it in front of them now," Virginia said, motioning to the snacks.

But putting fruits and vegetables in front of Wells hadn't yet proven particularly effective. Wells just bought junk food when he was out with his friends, returning home in the late afternoons and sneaking it into his room. When Virginia found out about Wells's secret stash of treats, she tried to instate new boundaries. "I said, 'You can have it outside of your room and just put it in a bowl, but I'm not going to let this be *in* your room.'"

But the next week came and Wells did it again, hiding a half-eaten bag of cookies in his nightstand. Wells's stubbornness tested Virginia, who found it hard not to fixate on what she deemed her personal failing as a mother. Tormented by his secrecy, she waffled on how best to approach the situation. Perhaps she could ask their pediatrician to intervene. Or she could leave Wells to his own devices and hope for the best.

Other affluent moms struggled with similar questions of how and how much to control their kids. Some even stressed about whether they were *over*controlling their children. Virginia was concerned that her continuous nagging might eventually have a negative impact on Wells. Maybe all her supervision now was shortsighted and would impede his ability to self-regulate in the future. "I realize I'm just setting him up for hoarding and hiding," Virginia said. Then, throwing her hands up in the air, she sighed. "So I'm like, 'All right. You're in charge of you. I cannot be in charge of what you eat!'"

But Virginia and I both knew that she didn't really mean it—that she'd keep on trying to be in charge until the day her son moved out. As his mom, she couldn't help it. A lifetime of training and practice in physical cultivation wasn't so easily undone. Sure, that evening, Virginia was exasperated. But I had a feeling that, as she'd done dozens of times before, she'd pull herself out of bed the next morning with renewed gusto. Maybe she'd even come up with a different strategy or a novel trick to test out. Wells's diet and weight would continue to matter to Virginia because they augured how he'd fare in the future. And Wells's future well-being and success, Virginia knew, would be the ultimate grade she'd earn as a mom. She couldn't bear the thought of a failing one.

CHAPTER 20

Stacking Up

"How would you compare the way your family eats to other families?"

This was a question I asked every parent I met. I intentionally worded the question to be ambiguous and vague. I wanted it to be unclear whether I was referring to other families in their neighborhood, their country, or around the world. My goal was to see who parents chose to stack themselves up against.

Parents answered the question by discussing all kinds of other families. Some mentioned families they'd met through their kids' schools, church services, or neighborhood potlucks. A few mentioned members of their own extended families. Others mentioned families who did or did not share their socioeconomic, cultural, or racial backgrounds. And still others described hypothetical families who they only imagined ate a certain way.

Lower-income moms generally compared themselves to other lower-income families. Often they underscored that they were doing comparatively *better* than these families. These moms knew how I, someone with socioeconomic privilege, might see them—how I might try to put them in a box before even hearing their story. Aware of poverty's stereotypes and stigmas, they distanced themselves from the former and deflected the latter. They impressed upon me that while they might be poor, they were not *poor*-poor. They were not as poor as other families.

They were self-sufficient. Doing okay. They weren't leeches on public resources or "welfare queens." Most of the time, they had enough money to buy food. When that wasn't the case, they had others they could turn to for help: a sister, a cousin, a neighbor, or—if they were in dire straits—a food pantry. Some other families, they told me, didn't have that. Other families might be struggling and failing; they were struggling and getting by.

Lower-income moms strove to show me all the ways they were thriving and not just surviving. They wanted to underscore for me all they *had* rather than what they lacked. And it was true. They had a lot—deep bonds between immediate and extended family, strong ties to community members and organizations, grit and perseverance in the face of hardship, kind, curious, and clever children, and an enduring hope for the future. But convincingly telling the story of their success benefited from a point of comparison. It helped to show how others were failing. In this way, social comparison to worse-off families was a key downscaling strategy; even when things were difficult, moms could downscale their challenges by highlighting others'.

Kiara Bell, a single mom of four, taught me this. I met Kiara at her home on Veterans Day. Like most houses on the street, Kiara's was fenced in by a black steel gate. The windows and doors were lined with bars, and the hum of cars on the adjacent freeway was deafening. Her neighbors to both sides sat on their front porches, while down the street, kids lined up at a one-man taco stand.

For the past two decades, Kiara had worked at a public elementary-school cafeteria. "I'm what you call a lunch lady," she said with a laugh as we sat down at her kitchen table and she kicked off her fuzzy zebra slippers. Kiara had curly short black hair, a broad face, and thick-framed tortoiseshell glasses that slipped down the bridge of her nose as she talked.

The steady income from working forty hours a week for twelve dollars an hour helped Kiara pay the rent on her nine-hundred-square-foot, two-bedroom house. Kiara's family was one of the few who had both qualified for and secured public housing. Her housing vouchers covered five hundred dollars of her fifteen-hundred-dollar monthly rent. After shelling out the remaining thousand each month, she used the rest of her income to feed, clothe, and care for her children.

"I think the more the economy gettin' higher, the more they think food is supposed to get higher too," Kiara told me, taking a sip of water from a tall green thermos. "A gallon of milk is almost five dollars, and I have four girls that drink milk. It's just crazy."

But pricey as food was, Kiara felt blessed by the support system that kept her kids fed and happy. Every month, she gave her grandmother, a retired school-bus driver, money to grocery shop for the entire family. The evening we met, like most evenings, Kiara would walk her kids over to her grandma's for dinner at five thirty. "We basically don't eat here," Kiara said, tapping the kitchen table with her index finger. "We eat at my grandmother's house."

Kiara, her aunt, and her brother all gave her grandmother money to feed the entire family. Kiara shared with her a SNAP debit card as well as an extra hundred dollars for food. Kiara knew that if it were just on her to feed the kids, she'd probably come up short. Even with the federal assistance, four girls with four growling stomachs and four growing bodies meant that food generally disappeared as quickly as it entered her house. But with everyone contributing, they rarely went hungry. "There's a lot of us eating together, you know?" Kiara said, peering out the window toward the freeway. "But it's a lot of us pitchin' in too."

Other families got by this way too, leveraging familial support to create their own informal safety net. When Kiara had more to contribute to the family's collective food budget, as happened some months, she did. Other months, when the kids' school supplies and an unexpected car-repair bill set her back, she leaned on her family to cover her share. The net was built on reciprocity and trust. Kiara knew it would be there to catch and cushion her if and when she fell.

But she knew other single moms with no safety net, formal or informal. She knew moms who were at the food pantry every *week* rather than every month or two. She knew moms who worked so many shifts they rarely sat down with their kids for a meal. She knew moms who would have qualified for all the help she got, but they were undocumented, so they had no housing vouchers, no SNAP funds, and no Medicaid. When Kiara thought of these moms, she knew she was doing okay.

Even though I had met Kiara outside a food bank—she was lined up along with dozens of other parents for a Thanksgiving food drive—Kiara was sure that her family was doing better than most. "I work for the school district, so I know a lot of babies come to school hungry, you know?" Kiara said, checking her nails for chips. Her job gave her firsthand exposure to just how bad things could get. Parents dropped their kids off at school with empty stomachs. Most of those kids had to eat the school breakfasts and lunches that she prepared, which were bland or unappetizing. Some kids wouldn't eat them even if they were starving.

But that, she reminded herself, was not her kids' situation. Her daughters never went to school hungry. And on days off, they always had food to eat at home. "Some babies is not gonna eat today 'cause school's not in," Kiara told me, her eyes widening. "Like, if it's vacation, what they gonna eat when they's on vacation? That's not fair for babies to come to school hungry." This reality both frustrated Kiara and reinforced her gratitude that she wasn't in that position. She could always manage to buy her kids food they'd eat.

"A lot of families can't afford food," Kiara told me. "If somebody has a lot of kids, they be hungry."

Although Kiara may not have deemed four kids a lot, to me, it didn't seem like *few* kids. It seemed like a good number of mouths to feed on a single income. It seemed, given the rising price of food and her daughters' growing appetites, stressful. It seemed, from what Kiara had shared, challenging.

But Kiara must have been imagining more kids—maybe five, six, or even seven kids. Families of that size were likely on her mind when she highlighted her lack of challenges when it came to feeding her family.

"Thank God for that!" She laughed. "No challenges, no. I have a lot of support. Even if I did, I have a lot of support so I wouldn't even have those challenges. Some people don't have that, so thank God for that. I won't have any of those challenges."

Even though Kiara felt like she was barely paying all the bills each month, she could downscale—even bury—her own struggles by summoning others' forward. She could stack her situation up against other families who were in even harder situations to assure herself that she was doing just fine. Kiara thought about unhoused people, people without extended family, people without stable jobs. "People that's living on streets that's homeless," she said. "They have challenges. And some people don't have—can't provide for their children.

"But"—she looked me in the eye—"I don't have those."

One morning a week after the utility bill was due, the water in Nyah's home was shut off. When I arrived in the early afternoon, Mariah and Natasha were visibly frustrated. Natasha sat on the garage sofa pouting, and Mariah headed out to meet friends, not saying goodbye to her mom as she strolled down the driveway. Nyah was irritated too but felt like the girls were being a bit dramatic. Nyah pointed out that they still had a roof over their heads, which was "better than a lot of other people," even if they couldn't take a shower that day.

"Some people don't have that," she reminded her daughters.

Nyah was often making these kinds of comments, putting things in perspective for Mariah and Natasha. She nudged them to remember how lucky they were to have everything they had: a microwave, two TVs, their own rooms. Back in Georgia, Nyah and her siblings had grown up "one on top of the other." By comparison, she was raising her kids in a mansion.

When Nyah picked up a thirty-six-pack of extra-soft toilet paper—the plush kind—on sale one afternoon, she told the girls they should appreciate the fact that they had toilet paper to begin with. On top of that, they could now enjoy the non-scratchy kind for a month. One morning, Mariah complained there was nothing to eat, but Nyah wasn't having it. Some people had literally nothing to eat at home, Nyah explained to her daughter. "We have a whole freezer full of meat in the garage," Nyah reminded her. "You go pick something out."

But as much as Nyah worked to assure the girls that all was well, she didn't really believe that they were in a good spot. I didn't need to read between the lines to see that. When she wasn't trying to put a positive spin on the situation, Nyah opened up often about how she felt down and depleted, how others didn't know her struggles, and how she was never sure if next month was the month in which she would finally receive the eviction notice she felt was coming down the line.

Yet, amid those worries, Nyah found the ability to buoy herself in moments by looking around at other families. Many other families she knew were also struggling or even worse off. Some lacked toilet paper or food to eat—problems she didn't face. Nyah always had a square to tear off or a chicken to defrost.

Lower-income moms' strategy of using other moms who were in worse shape as their basis of comparison was effective on different levels. It helped bolster their and their children's spirits under challenging circumstances. It also enabled moms to feel better about the particulars of their kids' diets. If other families weren't able to afford vegetables or meat, then getting kids to eat some of those was winning. What's more, if other families were barely able to feed their kids, then feeding kids *period* was a success.

The point is that even if their kids weren't the healthiest eaters, moms could use social comparison to find something about their diets to feel better—even good—about. For instance, some moms beamed with pride about their kids' adventurous tastes, highlighting the advantages of not having "picky eaters." Other moms underscored that their kids didn't want to watch TV when they ate or were eager to help with cooking. Finally, some moms focused on how their kids were doing better overall than their peers, their diets aside. This was the approach Faye Bautista, a single Filipina mom, took. Even though her sixteen-year-old daughter, Melanie, was eating fast food every evening, Faye knew she was still doing better than her peers.

"I see other children," Faye told me, "they do different things, like prostitute or something like that. But she's really good. I really admire her for that, and I thank her for that."

Wealthier moms also looked around to get a sense of how they were doing dietarily. But while observing other families helped lower-income moms feel better about their situations, doing the exact same thing had the opposite effect on their more affluent counterparts.

Social comparison only heightened affluent moms' anxiety and fueled their upscaling. When these moms observed their neighbors, colleagues, and fellow PTA members, they found proof that they could be doing better. Even moms' understanding of their relative privilege did little to reassure them. Some spoke about the challenges they knew food-insecure families faced or identified the fact that their kids didn't rely on school meals as a privilege. They expressed gratitude that they didn't have to worry about the price of food and about food deserts. Many knew about raging inequality in America. Still, acknowledging their privilege generally wasn't enough to put their situation into perspective for them.

This was never clearer to me than at the Halloween party I attended with Julie and Jane Cain. I met Julie at home on Halloween afternoon. As she and I were catching up at the kitchen island, Jane came downstairs from her room dressed in a black-and-white cow onesie. Pulling up a stool at the counter, she told me that we were going to the McGregors' house that night because they had a huge place that was good for hosting people.

"Our house isn't really good for parties." Jane sighed, grabbing a handful of candy corn out of a communal glass bowl. "We don't really have a backyard." I glanced out the kitchen window at the Cains' backyard; they had a deck with a grill and a giant trampoline. As I transferred the homemade meatballs Julie had prepared into a Tupperware container to bring to the party, I couldn't help picturing Dana's eight-hundred-square-foot apartment and Nyah's four-foot-wide gravel backyard.

Jane was doing a familiar dance, stacking her situation up against others'. I'd seen Julie do this too. Just the other afternoon, Julie and I had chatted about the nutritionist they'd hired to help Jane. Julie was encouraged by Jane's progress, but she still felt that her daughter wasn't where she should be. "I think other kids her age have this figured out," Julie had lamented as she washed a Gala apple in the sink. Julie dried the apple and placed it next to a sandwich-size Ziploc bag of fat-free popcorn. These, she told me, were Jane's after-school snacks for tomorrow.

Halloween afternoon, with the meatballs ready and the sun beginning to set, the three of us headed to the party. I followed Julie and Jane in my car on the ten-minute drive to the McGregors' calm, tree-lined residential street. The McGregors had decked both the inside and the outside of their two-story home for the occasion. There was a small, creepy clown by the front steps and a ghost hanging above the front door, and motion-sensor-activated skulls rolled along the winding brick path that connected the street to their home.

The party was largely concentrated on the sprawling front lawn, where teens and parents congregated in small groups. Most kids were in costume, some as giraffes and bunnies and others as Disney princesses and vampires. Moms wore fitted tees with pithy, holiday-themed messages like #PUMPKINEVERYTHING. Lawn chairs dotted the grass, and a long table wrapped in an orange tablecloth was covered in potluck contributions: Julie's meatballs, a vegetable lasagna, arugula salad, plain and pepperoni pizzas, a cheese platter, a bowl of sliced pineapple, mini–beef sliders, and homemade Halloween cupcakes.

As Jane joined her friends on the lawn, I followed Julie into the house and back to the kitchen. There, moms were filling sparkly tumblers with cocktails of vodka and blood-orange Italian soda. Lisa McGregor showed Julie the wheatgrass shot that she had been giving her daughter Melissa every day for the past month.

"What's that for?" Julie asked. Lisa explained that the shot was good for Melissa's immunity. Then, pointing to the handle of vodka on the counter, she said teasingly to Julie, "I know what you use for immunity!" Julie grinned, sipping her chilled cocktail through a straw.

The first twenty minutes of the party, I stuck out like a sore thumb. What was this twenty-something-year-old woman without children doing at a high-school Halloween party? No one knew who I was, and scribbling observations into my notebook wasn't helping me blend in. But that quickly changed. Within the hour, word got out that I was a researcher studying families and food, and I went from an awkward, uninvited intruder to a cameo-making celebrity. In droves, moms approached me to bare their souls. They shared how much they cared about healthy eating and how challenging it was to, as Lisa put it, "get it right." Some moms wanted me to understand the dietary principles or rules they followed, and others shared their go-to quick, easy, and healthy dinners. A few mentioned the vegetable gardens they were planting in their backyards or the cleanses they'd tried. Many brought up the absence of fast food from their own and their kids' diets.

And yet, a deep, palpable anxiety permeated these moms' boasting. Their feelings of pride seemed remarkably fragile and precarious, fueled by worry and a self-imposed call to hustle. While demonstrating to me their commitment to healthy and nutritious eating, they seemed hungry to do more. A handful of moms asked me for my "expert advice." What did I think of soy? What about gluten? Was juice ever okay? Was it terrible if their kid ate apples but not broccoli?

Underlying all of these questions were clearly deeper, more existential ones. Moms were asking me: How could they do better? How could they *be* better?

"He refuses to eat anything green," one mom complained about her fifteen-year-old wrestling and soccer-playing son. "He thinks Jack in the Box is a well-rounded diet."

Another was frustrated by her daughters' volleyball coach, whom she saw as too lenient. He let the girls eat Burger King at sleepaway tournaments. "That can't be good for their game!" She laughed, then called her daughter Caroline over to meet me and share the details. "Tell Priya!" she implored Caroline.

After an hour of fielding moms' questions and concerns, I realized that all of this conversation with anxious moms was making *me* anxious. After politely excusing myself, I retreated to the first-floor bathroom for a breather. I closed the toilet seat, sat down on top, pulled out my notebook, and started writing.

Why do I feel so worried for these moms? I scribbled, pondering why their anxiety felt contagious. Their nervousness made me feel nervous. I didn't even have kids at the time, but in that moment, I felt myself already starting to worry about what I would eventually feed them! I thought about what it would be like to be constantly surrounded by this apprehensive—and guilt-inducing—discourse. None of the questions moms had asked me had easy answers, and many sparked even more questions. The more you asked, the more confused you became. Moms were spinning in circles looking for a simple solution to their dietary woes.

Julie's social world consisted largely of the moms I'd met tonight. These were moms who, like Julie, were deeply invested in what their families ate. It made sense that they talked among themselves, bounced ideas around, and motivated one another. But I also saw how being in proximity to other moms made it hard not to discuss and compare. As moms gathered and chatted, as they evaluated one another's potluck contributions and observed other kids' consumption, they dug themselves deeper and deeper into worry. Their stress levels, significant already, seemed to soar to even greater heights.

Only a handful of lower-income moms said that working full-time made it extra-challenging to eat healthy, perhaps because few considered there to be an alternative. Full-time employment was a necessity, not a choice. But many working middle- and higher-income moms saw their jobs as major barriers. They perceived families with stay-at-home moms as better able to pull off the diets they aspired to. Empowered, progressive, and tenacious as they were professionally, they nonetheless felt a gnawing guilt that their desire, decision, or need to work undermined their maternal duty to feed.

Lori Galvez, a human resources director and mom of three, felt the frustration of a frenzied life. She also knew for certain that stay-at-home moms had it easier. A career-driven straight shooter, Lori worked fifty-hour weeks at a large nonprofit, spending ninety minutes in the car commuting every day. The afternoon I met Lori in her office for a "working lunch," she wore thick beige-framed glasses and a thin barrette pinning her wavy black hair to the side.

"I always feel guilty because I'm a working mom," Lori confessed, taking a sip of coffee. What she sacrificed by being a working mom, she felt, was the quality of her kids' diets. "I feel like the children don't get their three square meals like [the kids of] a lot of moms that don't work. I know a lot of them. I'm involved in the high school's performing-arts boosters and some of the other organizations at the high school. Most of those moms don't work or they work part-time. So the children get a breakfast in the morning, and their mom makes them lunch, and then they come home to a dinner at like five thirty."

This, Lori said with a laugh, was not her situation. Often, her three kids were responsible for figuring out their own lunches. "Winging it" for dinner was typical. While Lori loved her job and understood the inevitable trade-off of preparing nightly dinners from scratch in exchange for pursuing a high-powered career, acknowledging this trade-off seemed to do little to assuage her guilt. Rather than work through or reject the guilt, Lori accepted it, even indulged it. In some ways, it seemed like she owned it. She admitted to always feeling guilty, an experience that wore her down and made trying to manage her kids' diets feel like a losing battle.

Lori had countless examples of the ways that stay-at-home moms were doing better by their kids. Take grocery shopping, for instance. These moms, she explained, had all the time in the world to shop at different supermarkets, farmers' markets, and delicatessens. They could exercise creativity and ingenuity in ways Lori couldn't because she was behind a desk fifty hours a week. Worst of all, Lori feared that her kids' palates weren't developing like their peers'. "I mean, I barely got them eating hummus. That was, like, a big thing!" Lori laughed. But as proud as she was of her kids' acceptance of ground chickpeas,

Lori didn't have the bandwidth to make that kind of headway with other foods she would have liked to see them eating.

"I've talked to a lot of children nowadays that are getting more and more into a lot more vegetables." Lori sighed. "But I don't think my children eat as many vegetables as they should."

The power of social comparison really hit me when I met stay-at-home moms—the objects of Lori's nutritional envy—who also compared themselves to others and emerged feeling inadequate. Emma Romero, a stay-at-home mom of two, helped me see this. I met Emma one blustery evening at a public high school's PTA meeting. Emma, the PTA president, had a light brown, shoulder-length bob and a warm, bubbly personality.

"I do a lot of cooking," Emma told me as we cozied into a coffee shop's corner booth one morning the following week. Emma nibbled on her egg-white-and-spinach panini while I inhaled a bear claw pastry far less gracefully.

"Food's important to me," she said, "and I try to make sure it's filling emotionally and physically." Many weekdays, Emma mulled over, shopped for, prepped, and cooked food. While Emma felt strongly about healthy eating, she was happy to make her sons' favorite dishes as long as they met her desired ratios of vegetables, starches, and proteins. Emma cooked meals like fajitas, tortellini, turkey burgers, and salmon.

Emma also obliged their cravings for sweets, but on her own terms. When her sons requested cookies, Emma avoided the supermarket ones. "I don't like to buy those because they have trans fats," she explained. "And that's one of the reasons I like to bake. I know it's probably too much sugar but at least I know the ingredients, there are no preservatives, and at least, if they're getting something homemade sweet, it's better than buying something sweet."

Most recently, Emma had made a lemon pound cake and chewy maple cookies. So reliably did Emma bake that her sons came to expect homemade treats when they got home from school. "They feel neglected if there aren't cookies in the cookie jar!" Emma chuckled, taking a bite of her sandwich.

From my vantage point, Emma was the envy of all moms. She was doing what most said they wanted to do. She had the homemade meals, the organic fruits and veggies, the limitless time, the ample money, the white-cabinet kitchen, and the cooking know-how. *I've found her,* I thought, *the intensive mother herself.*

But even Emma was overcome by those familiar pangs of guilt. Even she felt that she wasn't doing as well as she could by her kids. With each passing year, Emma found new things to worry about. The day we met, she was newly frustrated by the fact that her kids weren't getting enough vegetables. The challenge was that with all the calories they were burning in after-school sports and their growing bodies, they wanted more filling foods that Emma knew were less healthy.

"I really need to push more vegetables and make sure they get the protein they need." She sighed, shaking her head. "I don't think I'm as good as I should be at it."

It certainly wasn't for a lack of effort on Emma's part that the boys weren't eating plates of greens. Emma made sure there were vegetables with every meal. She snuck them into casseroles and scrambled them into eggs. But she also turned to bread and pasta to fill them up when broccoli and carrots wouldn't. "I think I try," she reassured herself, "but [with] the stuff they like and the amount of food they need to eat, I feel like it's hard. I think that's my concern now. For them to be healthy and get the nutrition they need but still feel full."

When Emma looked around, she saw other mothers who were better at sticking to their guns when it came to their kids' diets. There were also moms who cooked more often, who whipped up more dishes from scratch, who packed nicer lunches, or who got their kids to stop pleading for soda.

"One friend," Emma told me, clearly envious, "she's really

just disciplined to begin with. She bakes but she bakes healthy
muffins and that kind of stuff but healthier than my chocolate
chip cookies. And they cook every night, every week, and really
only go out for birthdays, go out to eat." While Emma's oven-
baked sea bass and banana bread might have been the envy of
moms like Lori, Emma herself thought that she did not measure
up. For her, as for many moms, the well of reasons to feel less-
than was bottomless.

Emma was on my mind the next evening as I sat at my
kitchen counter jotting down some thoughts from our conversation. *Privilege has an irony to it,* I wrote. *I started off thinking that
affluent moms must have it so easy with food. What do they have to
worry about? But now I'm wondering if they're the most stressed of all.*

But when I stepped back and took a bird's-eye view, I realized that that assessment wasn't quite right; almost every mom
I'd met—rich or poor, Black or white, single or married—was
stressed. No mom believed that she was doing a good enough
job, and every mom felt the sting of falling short. Even if moms
used different emotion-work strategies for navigating those feelings of inadequacy, the fact that most moms had to use *any* strategy at all to save face and manage their self-worth pointed
toward the larger and more insidious structural problem: moms
were up against impossible standards but had little in the way of
support to give them a fighting chance. While moms felt like
they were failing their families, the more I observed their struggles, the more clearly and deeply I understood that it was actually society that was failing them.

PART V

Conclusion

Here I am, suspended
between the sidewalk and twilight,
the sky dimming so fast it seems alive.
What if you felt the invisible
tug between you and everything?

— Ellen Bass, "The World Has Need of You"

CHAPTER 21

Windfall

"Three hundred dollars goes a long way," Nyah said with a smile as I handed her a stiff white envelope with that amount of cash inside. It was a warm August afternoon, and we were standing by my car at the end of her driveway. I was giving Nyah the compensation for allowing me to observe her family. At the outset of my research, after consulting with advisers and colleagues, I had decided to pay families sixty dollars for interviews and three hundred for observations. The latter was enough for families to buy something special but not so large that it would coerce them into participating if they didn't want to. I offered families the option of receiving the money in installments throughout observations or all at once when my research was over. Every family chose to receive the full sum at the very end.[1]

I asked Nyah, Dana, Renata, and Julie to each keep track of how they spent the three hundred dollars. My interest was in understanding how a small windfall of cash might affect families' diets, particularly Nyah's and Dana's. Would moms put the money toward food purchases? Would they buy fruits and vegetables with it? Or would they devote it to other purposes, like covering rent, paying off a medical bill, or loaning it to a family member in need? So that moms wouldn't feel compelled to put the money toward a particular use, I reiterated to them multiple times that it didn't matter to me how they spent it. Based on what I later learned about where they each directed the money, I feel confident that they believed me.

As I considered how Nyah, Dana, Renata, and Julie would put the cash to use, I thought a lot about the food-access argument. I thought about how much healthy food's price and proximity shaped their families' diets. Proximity had never been a huge concern for any of these families, as none lived far from a supermarket. But price, especially to Nyah and Dana and somewhat to Renata, was a concern. With three hundred dollars, a lower-income family would temporarily be able to access healthy food. Three hundred dollars could pay for ten—maybe even twenty—nutritious meals. It could cover the cost of whole, organic foods and raw ingredients. If price was *the* primary barrier to healthy eating, then for at least the next week or two, a few hundred dollars should reduce that barrier.

Nyah took the sealed envelope in one hand and extended the other to shake mine. In light of how much time we'd spent together, the gesture felt oddly formal.

"Seriously, Priya, thank you," she said, leaning in to hug me. I wrapped my arm around her shoulder and explained, smiling, that she wasn't completely rid of me yet. Nyah's eyes opened wide, as they did when she was a little surprised. Then she laughed. "I know, I know, I'll be seein' ya," she said as she turned to walk back up the driveway. "Text me!" Then she disappeared through the front door.

Exactly a week later, I did. The next day, I was back in Nyah's living room crashing her and Mariah's movie marathon. In the center of the room was a queen-size air mattress covered in a white sheet and blue comforter that Nyah had been sleeping on the past three nights while Marcus's daughter was in town. I hadn't seen them watch TV inside before (we were usually out in Nyah's garage), but Nyah explained that her cable had been shut off a few days ago. Luckily, she could still watch one of her many pirated DVDs without paying a dime.

"I'm hiding my anxiety well." Nyah sighed, fast-forwarding through an episode of *Judge Judy*. "But it's through the roof right now with these bills."

Nyah broke down how she'd spent the three hundred dollars. First, she had decided to split it equally among herself and her daughters. That, I learned, had always been the plan. She kept a hundred dollars for herself and gave Mariah and Natasha each a hundred.

Wow, I thought. This was a woman I had once seen haggle with a cell phone agent to get a dollar off her phone bill, and she had just taken two hundred dollars and gifted it to her daughters to spend however they wanted. That money could have gone to all the bills that were giving Nyah anxiety attacks. It could have gone to the supermarket and a week's worth of healthy meals. It could have gone to the car's AC, months of cable, two cell phone bills, or the year's school supplies.

But Nyah didn't put that two hundred dollars toward any of that. She put it toward something bigger—something monumental, in fact. In giving Mariah and Natasha that money, Nyah gifted her kids "the best week of the entire summer," she said.

"That money put them in the driver's seat," Nyah told me as she grabbed a handful of pistachios from an orange bowl on the coffee table. The girls had gotten a glimpse of the summer they'd hoped for, one where they could do what they wanted. For a moment, they didn't have to ration or share. They didn't have to ask or plead. They didn't have to hear their mom say no.

They went to the mall to buy the clothes they coveted and the treats they wanted. At the mall, Mariah had spent forty dollars on a jean skirt and three tank tops. Then she'd bought two pizzas from Little Caesars for eleven dollars and gifted everyone in the family ice cream from the ice cream truck for ten dollars.

At a convenience store, Natasha had bought herself two hot fries and a blue Powerade for twelve bucks and burritos and sodas for the family for fourteen. She spent another fourteen dollars on ice cream over a week and gave Marcus ten dollars for gas. She went to the mall to buy clothes, but she got McDonald's and Mrs. Fields instead for ten bucks. Nyah told me that Natasha still had around thirty dollars left.

"And what about you?" I asked Nyah, reaching for some pistachios myself.

Nyah had used sixty of her one hundred dollars to pay off a utilities bill. She then put twenty dollars' worth of gas in the car. With the remaining twenty bucks, she bought herself some things she'd wanted: an eighteen-pack of beer and a bag of Doritos.

In the end, while some of Nyah's three hundred dollars had gone to paying the bills that kept her up at night, most of it had gone elsewhere—toward her daughters' and her own small pleasures. I tried to be surprised, but I wasn't. I wasn't surprised because what Nyah and I both knew was that once that money ran out, she was still going to be poor. Three hundred dollars wasn't going to substantively change anything in the long run about Nyah's circumstances. But for that week, instead of having to say no to her daughters and herself, Nyah had the rare opportunity to say yes. And for Nyah, that was worth far more than a week—or even two—of healthy meals.

Nyah's spending drove home the fact that for many families, small financial influxes would probably move the needle very little nutritionally. The exception was families who could not afford food at all to start; these families would undoubtedly use the money to feed their kids and themselves. But even for families like Nyah's, those who were far below the poverty line, who suffered from food insecurity, and who didn't always make rent each month, money was still better spent on their kids' happiness than on improving families' nutritional intake.

This was made even clearer to me when I learned that Dana had spent the money similarly, splitting it equally among herself and her daughters. Madison and Paige spent their money like Mariah and Natasha had, enjoying new clothes and food. With her hundred dollars, Dana got a haircut and extensions. With the remaining money, she took Madison out to dinner at their favorite sushi restaurant, splitting two rolls for twelve dollars and covering the tax and tip herself.

"Priya can come back and do more research," Madison said the evening I returned to check on the Williamses, a big grin sweeping across her face. "I want to get some more clothes."

I gave Julie her compensation on the afternoon of Halloween before I accompanied her and Jane to the neighborhood Halloween party. I'd held a big bag of pumpkin-shaped Reese's Peanut Butter Cups in one hand and rung the doorbell with the other. Julie greeted me in boot-cut jeans and a light gray Halloween T-shirt. She seemed a bit exasperated as she ran around the house gathering things for the party. I found Jane where she usually was, sitting at the kitchen counter playing on her phone. On the stove top were snacks and dishes for the party. A bag of mixed mini–candy bars lay next to a stack of napkins that each read DRINK UP, WITCHES! To the left I spotted a tray of mini-muffins with candy corn.

"Jane baked those," Julie told me. "We also have meatballs in the slow cooker."

When Jane headed upstairs to get her costume on, Julie took a seat at the counter and started texting. I knew the kids would come back any minute, so I handed her the envelope with the money. A warm smile shot across Julie's face.

"Ohhh, lovely!" she exclaimed, taking the envelope from me. "We will just put that in a safe spot, where nobody knows about it but me!" Julie laughed as she tucked the envelope into the front pocket of her purse. "Okay, perfect, thank you," she continued. I felt a bit dumbfounded. I had known that Julie didn't need the money, but it never occurred to me that she would hide the payment aspect of the research from her family. While Nyah and Dana had both instantly shared the money with their children, Julie told me that she would keep it to get herself something special.

But later, when I texted Julie to find out how she had spent the money, she said that she hadn't actually kept it for herself at all. Like the other moms, she had put it directly toward her kids. *We spent the money on all things Jane for her birthday party,* Julie texted. *Food, decorations, drinks, dessert.* While Julie certainly didn't need the money to pay for Jane's birthday party, nor did she spend more on it than she would have otherwise, I was still struck by the fact that she chose, like Nyah and Dana, to direct her windfall of cash toward her children.

Renata was the last mom to receive the three hundred dollars. As I had with Nyah, Dana, and Julie, I felt sad to say goodbye to her. I had enjoyed the time I'd spent with Renata— prepping dinner, attending church services, participating in Renata and Amalia's mom-and-daughter dance classes, and watching reality-TV shows in the living room.

Renata and I sat side by side on the couch with our eyes glued to the latest episode of *America's Got Talent.* We were enjoying a dinner of Little Caesars pizza and a homemade salad when I handed Renata her envelope.

"Oh, wow, thank you so much," Renata said, standing up to grab her purse. Tucking the envelope into an interior pocket, she looked at me and smiled. "We really had a blast. The kids and I will miss you." When I explained to her that I'd follow up to see how she spent the money, she said that she had lots of ideas. I texted Renata a week later to inquire about her decision, and she told me that she'd purposefully delayed choosing how to spend it. *I stashed the envelope in my purse and I'm carrying it around until I decide,* she texted back.

I followed up with her again the next week, at which point

she'd made the call. Renata had brought the envelope to church and opened it up during the service. *Where should this money go?* she had asked God.

I decided it would be a great idea to use it towards Nico's East Coast Trip, she texted. *It's a Travel Program with his school to visit Washington DC, NY, and Boston. I will make a monthly payment towards my balance with this $300.* A few minutes later, she followed up. *This is a really great help! Thank you!*

I reflected on how the other three moms had spent the money, and Renata's choice seemed fitting. In one important way, it was consistent with Nyah, Dana, and Julie. Every mom put most, if not all, of the payment toward her children. That was telling in and of itself, a clear signal of moms' devotion to their children's happiness and well-being. But Nyah and Dana had spent the money quickly, as a windfall, treating their daughters to luxuries they couldn't otherwise afford. Julie had also treated her daughter to a luxury, but one that she could have afforded anyway. Renata's choice fell somewhere in the middle. Renata didn't need the money to survive, and she didn't need it for the well-being of her kids. But it certainly eased some stress in her life and let her breathe a little easier. For all the moms, the money offered a momentary means to provide. In doing so, it helped silence, if only for that moment, the voices that repeatedly echoed in the back of their minds—the ones that made them ask themselves whether they were indeed "good."

CHAPTER 22

Where We Go

When I was thirteen, a pair of foster siblings came to live with us. On a scorching August afternoon, a brother and sister arrived at our doorstep, an oversize backpack slung over each one's shoulder and a piece of luggage at each one's feet. Eleven-year-old Carla and her thirteen-year-old brother, Rodrigo, had weathered years of emotional and physical trauma from their father.[1] For the past four months, the two kids had lived largely on their own in the family's trailer. Eventually, the neighbors had called Child Protective Services, and the pair had ended up in our home.

Carla had long, jet-black hair that hit just above her waist. When she let out a boisterous giggle, her wide, genuine smile revealed a gap between her two front teeth. Rodrigo was a few inches taller than his sister with wavy, side-swept hair. The two, like most brothers and sisters, bickered and made each other laugh. They loved to swim in the pool and play tag. Late at night, I'd sometimes find them side by side on the living-room couch hours after the rest of the family had gone to bed. They'd be watching cartoons on TV, the sound barely audible. Occasionally, I joined them, the soft glow of the TV illuminating our faces.

Scarcity had left an impression on Carla, who started hoarding food the day she moved in with us. In the trailer, the siblings had quickly run out of things to eat. There often wasn't enough to go around, and they didn't know when someone might drop off more food. In our house, there was usually something to eat, even if it wasn't always what I wanted. Still, Carla would stuff boxes of cereal and bags of cookies into her dresser drawers under heaps of unfolded clothes. Sometimes I'd overhear her munching on them as I passed by her closed bedroom door. Other times, the snacks appeared during the late-night television sessions. Cross-legged on the couch, she'd grab a cookie directly out of the bag and toss it into her mouth as she laughed along with the cartoons. When Carla's stomach called for something heartier, she'd grab a can of Chef Boyardee from her personal pantry. I enjoyed watching her pop open a can, squirt a generous amount of hot sauce inside, and devour the cold tomato-sauce-coated raviolis with a spoon. My mom, upon seeing Carla's attachment to the pasta, loaded the cupboards with the red-labeled cans. There was enough in those cupboards for Carla to live on Chef Boyardee alone for at least a week. Carla stockpiled them under her bed anyway.

Food scarcity, I learned, can haunt you.

Thirty years later, I found myself stockpiling cans. It was late February 2020, the beginning of a global pandemic that would bring the world to a halt. The coronavirus was spreading swiftly; first detected in China, it had already ballooned in South Korea and Italy and would soon topple much of Europe, the United States, and Latin America. In March, to curb its spread, the San Francisco Bay Area issued an order for all residents to shelter in place. With important exceptions, the order required people to stay at—and, if possible, work from—home. Residents were advised to have a month's supply of food on hand.

Which is how my husband and I ended up at the supermarket one Saturday evening at eight o'clock to find the pasta aisle raided, a few boxes of fusilli flipped on their sides on the bottom shelf. I grabbed those boxes as well as other nonperishables like jars of tomato sauce, cans of soup, rice, couscous, and beans. The frozen fruits and vegetables were already sold out. I got two pints of ice cream and two frozen pizzas. In the produce aisle, I snatched enough to last ten days—two packs of mushrooms, three heads of broccoli, tomatoes, peppers, and oranges—aware of most fruits' and vegetables' disappointingly limited refrigerated life. I bought extras to blanch and freeze. Rounding out the trip, I grabbed five boxes of chocolate chip cookies.

Checking out, piling our hundreds of dollars' worth of purchases onto the conveyor belt, I thought about Nyah. This was how Nyah had always shopped. On the first day of each month, she'd head to the discount grocer and buy enough food to last the next thirty days; when she swiped her EBT card, she was always within a few dollars of her monthly allotment. She'd return to her kitchen to fill the refrigerator and restock the cupboards. The last week of every month, the fridge was empty except for rows of condiments that were never thrown out. She and the girls lived off of the cupboards and freezer.

I recalled the stress that pulsed through Nyah each time she reached the checkout. As the cashier rang the items up, each appearing with its price on the screen above the register, Nyah worried about whether she'd made the right choices. Was she getting everything that she, Mariah, and Natasha needed? If this was all they'd have that month, would it make them happy? Would it give them something to look forward to? Would they miss anything? Would it even last the whole month?

That evening in the supermarket, as I pulled out my credit card to pay, I asked myself similar questions. And I wondered how many people were, for the first time, asking them too. The barren pasta and grain aisles suggested there was widespread anxiety about quantity and satiety. The empty frozen-produce section hinted at concern about having something healthy. But the nearly empty ice cream section and the shopping carts piled high with muffins and cakes also suggested a desire to find comfort and pleasure during a difficult time.

These fears make sense during a pandemic. When a viral outbreak shakes the world to its core, it is understandable for people to fear food scarcity. It's perfectly reasonable to stockpile foods with longer shelf lives. Certain sacrifices—like substituting frozen produce for fresh—are to be expected. And it is completely fair to prioritize satiating foods over healthier ones, because food provides a much-needed source of comfort for weathering hardship.

And yet, for millions of Americans, these trade-offs are a daily reality, pandemic or not. Our country didn't need a viral outbreak to create a context wherein far too many people's concerns about the quantity, quality, healthiness, cost, and purpose of food are rational and legitimate.

Every day in the United States, millions of people worry about the food they eat, and too few get the nutritious food they deserve. Many are hungry. Many sacrifice their own food intake to feed their children or pay their rent. Many use food to weather extreme adversity and buffer against scarcity. Others eat neither what they want nor what they need to feel healthy. Too many are rendered sick with chronic diseases by the food they consume. During the pandemic, as unemployment soared, so too did the demand for food banks and federal nutrition assistance. But even before this, the number of families forced to regularly line up outside food banks and access government funds to feed their families was unconscionably high. It has been unconscionably high for decades.

In one of the richest countries in the world, one that has more than enough food to feed every single family and where over half of produced food is dumped into landfills, this is a disgrace and a moral failing. Every family should be able to comfortably afford and access the food they need and, in addition, have the time, energy, and bandwidth to cook and consume it. No family should have to eat as if they are living through a pandemic that lasts their entire lifetimes. No family's consumption should be shaped by and subject to the scarcity, uncertainty, and anxiety that permeate so much of the American dietary experience.

These features of American eating also undermine the

American Dream. In the United States, we are told that we can become whatever we set our minds to—that everyone is entitled to a shot at success. But success is possible only when we consistently and dependably have nutritious food to eat. We deserve to eat and feed our families real food—healthy food—that keeps our bodies fueled and flourishing. We deserve to consume a diet that promotes our health rather than undermines it. But today, far too many Americans are living under circumstances that make getting what they deserve unlikely, if not impossible.

When I began the research for this book, common wisdom held that unequal food access was largely responsible for widespread nutritional inequality. Food deserts were supposedly to blame for low-income families' low-quality diets. Scholars and foodies alike argued that by increasing families' proximity to healthy food, kids' nutrition would improve. Over time, obesity rates would fall. The dietary gap would close. The food-access argument was popular in part because it implied a straightforward—not to mention doable—course of action. If access was the problem, then the solution was staring us in the face: open more supermarkets in low-income communities.

But over the years, this solution unfortunately proved to be hardly any solution at all. One reason, families taught me, was that food access was just one of many issues that directly affected their diets. In fact, families' diets are profoundly influenced by a sweeping array of social justice issues. These diets are affected by families' broader contexts, including their neighborhoods, schools, housing, and jobs. Food-access reforms have fallen short of enabling a nutritious diet for all families because they haven't addressed how every one of these contextual factors affects the food families consume. The reality is that these factors—from where parents can afford to live to the jobs parents work—fundamentally shape what food *means* to families, which in turn shapes how families eat.

Because of the hidden power of food's meanings, I learned that improving families' access to nutritious food is only the starting point, not the solution, to ensuring nutritional equity. Food access is a necessary but insufficient prerequisite. Reducing nutritional inequality will demand more than making fruits and vegetables widely available and affordable. It will require providing Americans with the financial, social, and emotional resources to make a nutritious diet realistic.

Most moms I met desired the same things for their kids. Moms wanted children to eat healthy, thrive, and be happy. Moms also shared overlapping ideas about what it would take to make that happen. But for most, insufficient resources rendered those aspirations unachievable. Whether it was too little money, not enough time, unpredictable work hours, absent social support, unstable housing, more pressing needs, or a lack of other comforts, trying to provide the ideal balance of nutritious foods was, for most mothers, akin to swimming upstream.

Moms also showed me that access to healthy food is about more than geography and finances. Access to healthy food means being able to live a life with resources and supports that make a nutritious diet the default, not the exception. Access to healthy food means not having to fight—to constantly struggle—to eat the food you want and deserve. It is one thing to be able to find and afford a head of cauliflower. But it is another to *want* to buy that cauliflower, to *choose* to spend one's money on that cauliflower (at the expense of other purchases), to *have the time* and *know-how* to cook that cauliflower, and to *possess the patience* to weather one's child's complaints and pleas for macaroni and cheese and soldier on to feed that cauliflower to one's child. Only a handful of parents I met had all of these things. The vast majority didn't. Families' contexts determined whether they had access to and the money to buy cauliflower, and those same contexts also shaped whether buying cauliflower made any sense, given everything else going on.

We have the power to re-create our society as one wherein every family has enough nutritious food and the bandwidth to cook and eat it. But doing this will require, first, recognizing that a nutritious diet is not a privilege to be bestowed upon a worthy few but a fundamental human right to which every single person—rich or poor, Black, brown, or white—is entitled. For too long, we have assumed that only a narrow slice of society should and can lay claim to a nutritious diet. We have grown so used to a dietary environment saturated with processed foods rife with added sugar, sodium, and fat that we assume those to be the ingredients to which most are entitled, while affluent people, foodies, and "health freaks" have the precious means to choose otherwise. Certainly, processed treats can have their place. But they do not belong at the center of our diets. Making meaningful dietary improvements across society requires stating loudly and clearly this fundamental truth: every single one of us deserves the means to eat healthfully. Every single one of us deserves to eat food that meets our tastes, respects our unique and collective identities, and fosters our health.

We must also assume collective ownership for this human right. For too long, our country has placed the burden of eating healthy on individuals and families. That burden has often fallen on mothers. But there is no biological reason why food should be solely mothers' cognitive, emotional, and logistical responsibility to shoulder. As a society, we should consider foodwork—the labor of nourishing current and future generations—a cornerstone of American infrastructure. And rather than being deemed "women's work," these tasks should be distributed equitably and broadly to include fathers, partners, schools, and workplaces.[2]

In addition to burdening mothers with an enormous responsibility that should be shared instead, this country has long been deferential to the food industry's interests. It has been overly invested in a corporate-serving narrative of personal responsibility with no parallel requirement of social responsibility. This personal responsibility narrative—which underscores that individuals' diets and health are up to them alone—often resonates because of a broader ethos of American individualism as well as how individual our diets feel. Optimal health comes from discipline and disease from laziness, the narrative goes.

It is time not only to reject that rhetoric but to turn our gaze outward. Personal responsibility has never solved a public health problem or remedied an inequity. Food is no exception. Certainly, many of us could make small choices to eat differently. Many of the families I met had either done so or were trying to figure out how to eat more nutritiously with the resources they had. But, largely due to the structures implemented by the food industry and federal government, most felt like they were fighting an uphill battle—and losing.

Assuming a collective responsibility demands policy changes over personal ones. And food-specific policy reforms are an important place to start. For years, society has accepted federal nutrition-assistance programs and food banks as essential scaffolds that allow low-income families to eat. But these programs and institutions were designed to provide emergency relief, *not* to support daily life. What's more, food-assistance programs still remain underutilized.[3] Undocumented families are ineligible for programs like SNAP, and language barriers and government distrust can prevent qualifying immigrant families from accessing these benefits. We need real, concerted efforts to increase enrollment to ensure the broadest swath of society has access to this aid.[4] These programs must also move beyond reducing hunger and realize their potential to improve nutrition, which they currently do an inadequate job of.[5] As long as families are still stretching their personal and federal dollars to keep everyone fed, full, and happy, the quality of families' purchases may remain low. Families must feel financially empowered and capable of buying the nutritious foods they want and deserve.[6]

This means, first, expanding the amount of money that families receive in food assistance each month. At the time of the writing of this book, there are encouraging signs that food-assistance benefits may increase in a lasting way. The coronavirus pandemic and accompanying economic upheaval of 2020 sparked a hunger crisis in the United States, leading an additional 4.5 million Americans to enroll in SNAP. In response, in early 2021, the Biden administration accelerated a campaign of hunger relief that increased SNAP benefits by more than one billion dollars a month and set the stage for lasting expansions of food assistance. This is exciting because programs like SNAP and WIC will be most effective when they guarantee that families have enough food; removing concerns about hunger and satiety grants families the financial bandwidth to prioritize nutrition.

Introducing financial incentives to promote the purchase of nutritious foods can also aid in this. Incentive programs work by stretching federal-assistance dollars further when families purchase nutritious foods. Already, these incentive programs are being piloted in communities across the country. Double Up Food Bucks and Healthy Incentives Pilot programs incentivize fruit and vegetable purchases, the former by doubling allotments to purchase nutritious foods and the latter by offering a thirty-cent rebate for every SNAP dollar spent on fruits and vegetables. These incentives increase families' purchasing power and reduce the tough choices that families are often forced to make between a nutritious purchase and one that packs a higher caloric, emotional, or symbolic punch. They allow parents to buy nutritious foods while also granting them resources to indulge some of their kids' food requests. So far, the results suggest that these programs encourage more nutritious consumption.[7]

We must also expand and improve the National School Lunch Program and the School Breakfast Program, which serve free- and reduced-price lunches and breakfasts to low-income students across the country. Every day, thirty-one million children eat school meals; for some, these meals make up half of their daily calories.[8] But so many more children would benefit from access to free or subsidized meals during the school day. Indeed, a universal school-meal program—available to all students, regardless of family income—would help support children's nutritional intake, rectify socioeconomic and racial inequalities, and improve learning outcomes.[9] While universal school meals are common in many industrialized nations, the proposition has long been seen as radical in the United States and politically unfeasible, particularly in recent years under a Republican administration. But the coronavirus pandemic began to change that; incredible economic hardship, sudden school closures, and soaring rates of food insecurity put pressure on school districts to find creative ways to equitably feed more hungry children within highly constrained budgets. To support schools, the USDA began to offer federal waivers that reimbursed school districts for meals that were available to all students, regardless of income. This policy not only offered a lifeline to families but also began to lay the groundwork for a similar long-term solution. The universal school meal is an idea whose time may have finally come in America.

Alongside expanding the program to serve more children, the USDA needs to significantly improve the nutritional quality and aesthetic appeal of these meals. Corporate interests have long been and remain the biggest barrier to nutritious school meals. Because school meals fall under the jurisdiction of the Department of Agriculture, entities like the dairy lobby have an outsize influence on what goes on kids' plates. It is how school cafeterias end up overflowing with cheese pizza and cartons of chocolate milk. The Obama administration's Healthy, Hunger-Free Kids Act of 2010 took the biggest stride in recent history to improve school food. It updated nutrition standards to align with the *Dietary Guidelines for Americans,* upping the availability and portion sizes of fruits, vegetables, and whole grains, requiring kids to select a fruit or vegetable with each meal, establishing calorie ranges, removing trans fats, and limiting sodium levels.

Many of those improvements were rolled back under the Trump administration beginning in 2016, but we must continue to fight for higher-quality, nutritious school meals that not only nourish children but also teach kids about food, expose them to new ingredients, flavors, and dishes, and shape their understanding of food. Currently, school meals are blatantly homogenous, inadequately reflecting the diversity of students who eat them. Apart from the occasional taco, cafeteria fare is supposedly "American," featuring items like burgers and fries. But what if kids saw themselves reflected in school meals? What if the dishes schools served helped kids learn to appreciate a wider range of cultural cuisines? Just as food has the power to connect, school food can help cultivate kids' taste for different ingredients, spices, and dishes while fostering an appreciation of America's diverse culinary landscape. Schools could become powerful sites for nourishing and teaching kids all the ways to eat a nutritious diet. Schools could offer nutritious foods from all over the world, from aloo gobi to pho to paella. They could prepare meals that celebrate the traditions and dishes of the communities they serve. They could also provide and teach about ingredients that are globally shared; for instance, cafeterias could showcase all the different cultural variations of dumplings, such as samosas, *gyoza*, empanadas, *fufu*, and ravioli.

Increasing kids' access to healthy meals must be coupled with minimizing their exposure to junk food. This requires regulating the food industry, which currently spends almost two billion dollars a year on marketing to youth, targeting its least nutritious brands to Black and Latinx kids. The solution is to ban marketing to children, which is also the recommendation of every leading public health expert and organization that has taken this issue on. Currently, the only marketing regulation in schools is that companies cannot market items that don't meet school-nutrition standards. But this still allows companies to sell slightly healthier junk food in vending machines and snack shops and to market junk food through branded fundraisers, "educational" materials, incentives for teachers, and sponsorships.[10]

Banning marketing to children would benefit kids and parents. If kids weren't inundated with ads for unhealthy treats on TV, on their phones, and in schools, they would stop asking their parents for them nonstop. Moms wouldn't have to decide between saying no and risking a battle with their kids and saying yes and giving their kids something they don't want to.

Currently, corporations hide behind the guise of "helping" moms feed their kids. They promise moms ease, comfort, and convenience. They promise moms quiet, happy children. They promise moms the chance to be "good" by making their lives easier and getting their kids fed. They promise less sodium and fat and more whole grains and protein. They promise health. But apart from, perhaps, convenience, the industry does not deliver on any of these promises. In fact, it brings parents the exact opposite. It fosters nagging and begging. It prompts meltdowns and tantrums in the supermarket. It forces moms to sacrifice their preferences to keep kids quiet and content. It promotes lies about food's qualities and benefits.

It also increases maternal guilt, anxiety, and shame. Today, because feeding families largely remains moms' work, moms are the ones who primarily suffer from the food industry's power and reach. They are the ones who have to navigate their kids' preferences. They have to bear the weight of judgment—by society at large and internalized by themselves—for what goes into their kids' bodies. Corporations make moms harder on themselves than they already are by reinforcing the idea that moms alone are responsible for what their kids eat, all the while bombarding kids with ads for foods that deviate from the nutritious diets moms want them to eat.

Banning marketing to kids would give moms a fighting chance of being able to feed their kids what *they* want rather than what corporations push on them. Currently, only those families with the most money, time, and bandwidth have a shot at prevailing against the industry—and even those families often struggle and even fail. Protection from the food industry should be a right granted to all families, not a privilege reserved for the few.[11]

Food-specific reforms must be accompanied by sweeping structural reforms that materially better families' conditions. While increasing SNAP benefits and access to free and reduced-price school meals is an important expansion of the social safety net, the primary societal goal should be to invest so strongly in families that there is no need for these programs in the first place. A broad, societal investment in families means lifting parents out of poverty and offering them the opportunities they deserve to raise their children with a sense of self-worth and support. It means ensuring that every family has the financial, psychological, and emotional resources to feed themselves the way they desire and deserve. Poverty rates are higher in the U.S. than in other industrialized nations because we lack the policies to support those at risk of being poor. We need structural solutions that make it possible for all families to live with the security, stability, and dignity to which they are entitled. Key to these structural changes is tackling the underlying conditions that cement families in place at or below the poverty line.

The first condition is the lack of a living wage. Most low-income parents I met worked full-time, but for too many of them, the wage they made was simply not enough to predictably feed and provide for their children. That parents were working themselves to the bone to merely scrape by is unacceptable. A living wage would allow a parent to work one job instead of the two or three many hold today. It would grant parents a predictable, consistent income that would make a reliable monthly budget possible. It would give them hours back to spend grocery shopping and cooking; it would preserve precious time for them to spend with their kids and make positive, new memories with them. By giving parents more financial and temporal resources to invest in their children, a livable wage's impact on parents' sense of dignity would be as wide-reaching as its economic influence. Together, these positive changes would shift the symbolic meaning of junk food for lower-income parents. With more time and money to spend on other things for their kids, a bag of Doritos would go from being a potent symbol of love and care to being, well, just a bag of Doritos.

Beyond work, America must tackle housing, another underlying condition of poverty. America is in an affordable-housing crisis, as housing prices have outpaced wages and the affordable-housing supply falls drastically short of demand. California, where four out of five low-income households spend more than 30 percent of their income on rent, is one of the least affordable places to live. Most low-income families I met spent more than half of their income on rent, just like over a quarter of renters nationally do. There is also not enough federal assistance for housing; nationally, only one in five low-income households that need federal rental assistance receive it.[12]

Families I met who couldn't access federal assistance found housing solutions that came at a high financial, psychological, or emotional cost. These solutions demanded sacrifices that no parent should have to make. Parents rented spare rooms for their kids in shared apartments with kitchen cupboards padlocked to keep roommates from eating their food. Others doubled up with family and friends, lived in cars, crashed on living-room couches, or slept in bathtubs. Other parents paid market rates, which landed them in homes with unsafe or unsanitary conditions. I encountered bathrooms covered in mold, overrun with cockroaches, and echoing with the sounds of rats between the walls. I interviewed families that lived in neighborhoods with notoriously poor air quality and those that put up with leaky roofs and no hot water. The poor housing quality I witnessed has been shown to increase parents' stress and anxiety and damage kids' mental and physical health.[13] These parents also faced housing instability, including forced moves and evictions.[14] I met families who had weathered up to four evictions in the past few years. Each one of these moves was destabilizing for families, increasing their financial stress and stripping away the psychological and physical security of having a home. Parents who experience eviction suffer more material hardship, parenting stress, and maternal depression.[15]

Investing in affordable housing for all families makes both economic and nutritional sense. Unstable, unsafe, and over-priced housing zaps parents' resources for food, as they expend time, energy, and money struggling to keep a roof over their kids' heads. Conversely, better housing portends better nutrition for children; as households have to devote less of their income to housing expenses, their budget shares for food and other necessities increase.[16] They simply have more money with which to feed kids. When parents are worried about environmental toxins and eviction, they have less time and energy to focus on kids' diets. They must prioritize more pressing needs, like clean air and shelter. A stable, safe address means the ability to keep the same jobs and maintain kids' enrollment in the same schools. It can mean a shorter commute and more time at home. It means always having a kitchen to cook in and a fridge to store perishables. It means not wondering how, when, and with what money you will feed your children. It means a table around which to share meals with your children. It means stability and security, which increase the latitude to move nutritious eating up on parents' priority lists.

Finally, beyond poverty-focused policies, universal policies would benefit *all* American families and have positive, cascading effects on their diets. Industrialized nations with strong federal family policies offer paid family leave, paid sick and vacation leave, subsidized preschool, and universal health-care coverage.[17] In the United States, no such policies exist at the federal level, although as I write this book, there are signs that that may soon change. President Biden has recently proposed the American Families

Plan, part of a broader spending proposal to combat the economic downturn of the pandemic. In addition to offering universal free preschool, the plan would establish a nationally mandated paid parental, family, and personal-illness leave.[18]

The plan's proposed policies make sense because they account for the realities of modern parenthood and families' struggles to make ends meet. When parents can't afford to take leave without pay, they either don't take leave, take less leave than they need, or take leave and lose wages. Single mothers, especially of color, suffer the most without these safety-net provisions. Most low-income moms I met were single moms who did not receive child support. They were also entitled to zero paid leave with the birth of their children, had few sick days, and generally no vacation days. When a baby or family member needed caretaking, moms quit their jobs or reduced their work hours. When they were then no longer able to afford rent, some moved themselves and their kids in with a grandmother or aunt at best, into shelters or cars at worst. They experienced corrosive stress and anxiety about keeping a roof over their children's heads and their own two feet on the ground. Policies that help assure parental employment and income through tough times would help.

Together, structural wage and housing reforms could transform the contexts within which parents—and, in particular, moms—are raising and feeding their kids. It would lift them out of scarcity and into sufficiency. Remove the ongoing struggle and trauma of deprivation, and parents can worry less about children's safety and psychological health. Remove the destabilizations, stresses, and fears that characterize American poverty, and parents have the financial and emotional bandwidth to focus on other dimensions of their kids' well-being, like their diets, knowing full well that their kids are broadly okay. By granting families more financial security, less stress, and more time and bandwidth to care for loved ones, a tide of universal, family policies would help lift all boats.[19]

The point is simple: When parents are cared for by society, they can best support their kids. When our government and leaders support all individuals, no matter their circumstances, we each have a real chance to meaningfully care for ourselves and our loved ones.

The policy reforms and structural changes I laid out, along with others, will be key to reducing nutritional inequality and ensuring that all families have the means to consume a nutritious diet. But as we work collectively toward these changes, there is a role for each of us as individuals. It starts in the way that we talk about food. Our words have power. They can encourage empathy or judgment, understanding or critique. When we judge others for their food choices, we help build a more judgmental society. In contrast, when we consider what we would do in their shoes, we create a more compassionate one.

Together, we can shift the conversation around food and nutrition to assign less individual culpability and instead hold policy makers and corporations accountable. When confronted with negative portrayals of how families and kids eat, we always have a choice. We can dig in our heels and perpetuate a culture of individual judgment and blame, or we can pause to consider the larger influence of impossibly challenging contexts, parental pressures, inadequate social policies, and corporate interests.

This applies specifically to how we talk about mothers and food. The moms I met and my own experiences in motherhood showed me how widely reaching and deeply resonant society's critiques of moms can be. There is, apparently, no correct way to feed a child. Society reminds moms that no matter what they do, there is always something they should be doing better, from reducing their kids' sugar intake to expanding their palates to avoiding formula. Moms are expected to achieve the impossible: ward off a predatory food industry, prepare healthy home-made meals, and follow ever-evolving nutritional advice. On top of all that, they are expected to enjoy doing it! Moms are supposed to embrace being on the hook for their children's intake and accept responsibility for how that intake shapes their kids' bodies. Moms shouldn't mind that others use their kids as central sources of feedback about their maternal worth. What's more, moms should be thankful for the feedback, even though it is most often used to reveal to them their inadequacies and shortcomings.

This questionable and precarious gold standard of intensive mothering requires that moms keep striving to do more, to *be* more. It rewards a select few as laudable, while the vast majority can never be child-centered, labor-intensive, expert-guided, or emotionally absorbed enough. Moms of color and single and low-income moms suffer the most under the assumptions and prejudices built into our societal ideals of motherhood. These ideals add to the already heavy burdens these moms carry, as they must continually demonstrate that they are caring, committed providers, not the negligent, uncaring ones society generally casts them as.

That said, I was also struck by this simple truth: even moms who had the deck stacked in their favor often still felt like they were falling short. Before beginning this research, I expected to meet at least one mom who felt really good about how her family was eating. As I continued my interviews and observations, I kept waiting to meet her. *She's out there*, I told myself. She had to be.

But I never found this elusive mother, the one who truly appreciated and patted herself on the back for all the hard work she put in, the one who knew that she was doing an incredible job. Instead, my conversations with moms left me feeling disappointed and mystified. What does it say about our society that even the most privileged moms were generally riddled with stress and feelings of inadequacy about their kids' diets and their own worth as mothers?

These challenges also felt personal to moms, like something

they alone were battling and that was up to them as individuals to solve. Most moms were mired in intensive mothering's expectations and could not see the forest for the trees; they weren't aware that every other mom around them was fighting a similar fight and feeling like she was failing. But from where I was sitting, moms weren't the failures. Society had failed them.

If we as a society are to stop piling feelings of failure onto mothers, we have to unlearn what we have been socialized to believe about motherhood. Each of us individually can start by recognizing, appreciating, and supporting all of the hard work that mothers across society devote to nourishing their children. We can question the sexist, classist, and racist biases and assumptions that lead us to critique them so harshly. We can recognize that at the same time that American society has fallen short of supporting families' diets, it has encouraged us to judge others—and ourselves—unforgivingly for how we eat. And we can take steps to change that reality—to hold ourselves and others to a higher standard.

The point is: just because our country has long been this way does not mean its future is set in stone. Our nutritional problems are neither inevitable nor intractable. Together, we can chart the path toward remedying nutritional inequality in America, one grounded in understanding and empathy for individuals and families and accountability and action for the public and private sectors.

The future of our own and our children's health is at stake, and it depends on our ability to reimagine and reshape our country in a way that takes ownership for everyone's well-being. It hinges on our ability to collectively shoulder the responsibility not just for our own future but for our children's futures as well. Are we willing to do what it takes to ensure that families—*all* families—have the means to eat nutritiously? Nothing less than our collective health and well-being depend on our answer to that question.

About This Project

In the summer of 2013, I spent two months working in the nutrition policy department of the Washington, DC–based Center for Science in the Public Interest (CSPI), one of America's oldest and most powerful consumer advocacy groups promoting safer and healthier foods.[1] My primary job was to conduct research on checkout aisles.

"Checkout aisles?" friends and colleagues asked me, furrowing their brows. I nodded, agreeing that these seemed an unusual object of study. But for an organization interested in understanding all features of the American food environment, checkout aisles were worthy of investigation. For years, food and beverage corporations have strategically and unabashedly worked to bombard shoppers with low-cost, high-calorie, unhealthy treats at the end of their shopping trips. My responsibility that summer was to document how and with what temptations checkout aisles were luring consumers.

For two swampy months, I traveled around the District of Columbia visiting chain stores—including supermarkets, pharmacies, gas stations, and toy shops—to record in excruciating detail what they stocked in their checkout aisles. A clipboard in one hand and mechanical pencil in the other, I spent hours examining shelves of processed foods. I counted bags of chips and tallied cans of soda. I answered employees' inquiries about who I was and what I was doing. I got kicked out of Bed, Bath, and Beyond—twice.[2]

Researching checkout aisles expanded my understanding of the American food environment. It also gave me informal opportunities to observe people navigating it. I watched customers place last-minute Almond Joys on conveyor belts and nine-year-olds melt down at moms' refusal to buy them Twixes. I saw how the food industry preyed on consumers and left them feeling tempted, frustrated, and confused. That summer, when I wasn't standing in checkout lanes, I was reading about food in America. I started learning more and more about nutritional inequalities, which made it clear to me that not all consumers were equally positioned and privileged to push back against this industry.

I wanted to understand these inequalities' root causes.

At the time, most popular and scholarly commentary on nutritional inequality focused on financial and geographic food access, food deserts in particular. I was suspicious of this discourse's oversimplification of what I saw as an extremely complex topic. I believed that food access shaped people's diets in different ways, but I questioned whether food's price and proximity were the sole, or even primary, determinants of food choice. Rather, I suspected that these factors interacted with others to differently shape people's diets and fuel broader diet and health disparities.

When I returned to Stanford University in the fall of 2013, I began designing a research study to investigate, through interviews and observations, the facts and forces driving people's food choices. The negotiations and meltdowns I had witnessed at checkout aisles drew me to focus on parents. Parents had to navigate the food environment not only as eaters but as feeders.

Over the next two years, I interviewed one hundred sixty parents and kids and conducted two hundred hours of observations among families and in public schools. While the vast majority of these data did not make it into this book's pages, they vitally shaped everything that did.

Many parents I interviewed had kids from six months to twenty-five years old. But all were parents of at least one teenager. I decided to focus on families with teenagers, precisely because the teenage years are difficult ones nutritionally; kids' diets usually decrease in quality as they become teenagers. I wanted to see how parents and kids from all kinds of families navigated this challenging phase. In every family, I interviewed at least one parent and one teen and sometimes other family members too. Hearing different perspectives helped me grasp the push and pull of each generation on what was consumed and garner a fuller, more accurate picture of families' food patterns. I interviewed kids and parents separately, usually at home. Grant funding allowed me to compensate each family that participated in an interview with sixty dollars.

I spoke with a range of families that differed socioeconomically and ethno-racially, including roughly equal numbers of families from low, middle, and high socioeconomic backgrounds, as well as white, Black, Latinx, Asian, and multiracial families.[3] I made sure to speak with first- and second-generation families as well as those with deep roots in the United States; married, cohabiting, and single parents; and single- and double-earner families.[4] This variation allowed me to learn about as many different families' experiences as possible while also distilling common themes and shared experiences. It showed me how different types of resources and privileges are intimately entwined in people's food choices, sometimes in unexpected ways.

I began recruiting families for the research at Hillview Central High School, a public high school with short buildings and grassy knolls located on a quiet middle-class residential street in Silicon Valley. My plan was to find families to interview while observing students at the school. Hillview's student body was unusually socioeconomically diverse, which would facilitate recruiting a diverse group of families.

My doctoral mentor connected me with Nicola Vasquez, a

bubbly twenty-something Spanish and physical-education teacher with long black hair and an infectious smile. I visited Nicola at Hillview on a Friday morning and we toured the campus, meandering between security guards in golf carts and harried teachers wrangling clusters of students back into classrooms. Twenty minutes after Nicola shook my hand, she was convinced that Hillview was the right place for me to conduct my research.

"We should get you in to see Martin today," Nicola said. She led me to the principal's office, where I found myself face-to-face with the man himself. Martin Schnell, Hillview's new principal, was an endearingly gruff man with squinting eyes, thick, black-framed glasses, and a white goatee.

"Who are you and what do you want from me?" Martin looked up briefly, his brow furrowed, from a towering stack of papers on a cluttered desk as I stood motionless in his doorway. I eagerly delivered my spiel, hoping he wouldn't notice the quiver in my voice. I was a doctoral student, I explained, interested in researching how his students and their families ate. Martin, a new principal eager to make a name for himself, was into it.

"I could be the nutrition principal!" He chuckled before cuing me to leave by refocusing on his paperwork.

Three weeks later, I had secured approval for the research from Stanford's ethics review board, and Martin had obtained Hillview parents' permission.

"You'll always need to pick up a visitor pass in the front office when you come here," Martin informed me during one of our early meetings. But this formality soon disappeared, as I morphed quickly from a school visitor to a regular fixture. Over the next year, students and staff came to know me as a nonintrusive addition to the community. I found families to interview through teachers, staff, and students themselves. I attended PTA meetings and watched baseball games. I helped run the student store, a windowless room near the front office that sold Smart

Snacks and flavored water. Lunch ladies recognized me, as did student council members, sports coaches, and security guards. Some knew me by my real name but most warmly referred to me as the "nutrition lady" (despite my insistence that I was not a nutritionist).

After months at Hillview, I decided to expand my research beyond its campus to find a broader diversity of families. Hillview families were primarily middle- and high-income white families and low-income Latinx families. But I also wanted to speak with Black and Asian families, low-income white families, and high-income Latinx families.

My catchment area became the Bay Area in its entirety, and I found families through a variety of methods. I approached them in person at shopping malls, gyms, gas stations, pharmacies, and churches. I posted about my study on social media sites and professional listservs. I hung flyers at local grocers and community centers. I also used limited snowball sampling, meaning that families I interviewed referred me to other families.

Recruiting families in the community was not as easy as it was at Hillview. I was regularly turned down, stood up, and canceled on. I quickly discovered that I was an unessential addition to families' busy calendars. I learned to always confirm twenty-four hours before an interview and to carry an engaging book with me wherever I went in case I found myself waiting around for an hour or two.

Some families were simpler to recruit than others. Wealthy white and East and South Asian families went out of their way to participate. When my husband posted my recruitment pitch to his college alumni listserv, I received an onslaught of e-mail. For once, *I* was the one having to turn families down. But affluent Black and low-income Asian families were virtually impossible for me to recruit by myself. Historical legacies of exploitation and mistreatment by academics—medical researchers in particular—made members of these communities rightfully suspicious of participating. I built relationships with gatekeepers—trusted members—of these communities, who vouched for me and connected me to other families. Janae Lathrop, the initially wary mom I introduced in chapter 10, was one such gatekeeper. After our interview, Janae e-mailed her wider network of affluent Black mothers to let them know about my study. For the following two days, my in-box was flooded with interested moms reaching out to learn more about the research and find out how to participate.

Interviews are useful for learning about people's experiences, memories, meanings, perceptions, and judgments. But they also have their limits, subject as they are to people's filters and face-saving desires. Food in particular is a loaded, sensitive topic and therefore extra-challenging to discuss candidly. Emphasizing my sociological—not nutritional—focus to families was one way that I navigated these challenges. Once inside their homes, I typically began by defining my professional identity. "I'm a sociologist," I'd say with a smile. "*Not* a nutritionist."

Parents would often respond with theatrical sighs of relief. I made it clear that I didn't want to count their calories, nor was I invested in how healthy or unhealthy their diets were. It didn't matter to me if they drank sodas or ate brussels sprouts. But what they could help me understand, I explained, was how and why they ate the way they did. I was there to listen and learn. No detail was too small or too random, and there was no such thing as a right or wrong answer. Most important, I assured them they could speak honestly without fear of judgment. I took it as the highest compliment of the trust I'd built when parents said they'd been more honest with me about their diets than they were with their doctor.

Creating a nonjudgmental space was key to learning from families. Interviewing multiple family members also helped me better understand a family's food patterns. That parents' and kids' accounts generally aligned gave me confidence that I was getting a reasonably accurate view of how families ate. And when there were discrepancies between the stories, I returned to each family member to discuss and, if possible, resolve them.

I also modeled my desire for honesty and detail by asking open-ended questions that allowed families to talk at length. My probes delved into not only how families ate but also how they *thought* and *felt* about food. What role did food play in their lives? What meanings did it hold for them? And how did those meanings translate, if at all, into their food choices?

With all families, I explored the role of finances, culture, and convenience in shaping their diets. I also dug into the places they spent time and how those influenced their food choices. What was their neighborhood like? What shops and stores were nearby, and what was missing? What kind of food did they serve at work, church, and school? How did their friends and families eat, and what pressures did that exert on their own diets? With lower-income families, I explored their experiences with food insecurity, their participation in formal safety-net programs like SNAP and WIC, and how they cast their own informal safety net through food banks and social support. I inquired about parents' food histories: What kind of food had they grown up with and how had those experiences shaped the way they ate now, if at all? I talked to kids about how they ate not only with their families but also with their friends and classmates.

Still, I knew that no matter how much I tried to make the interview about families, who I was shaped what transpired between us. My identity opened certain doors and undoubtedly closed others in this research. Being a woman was beneficial—arguably crucial—since conducting interviews involved spending many hours alone with mothers and children. My gender helped moms feel comfortable leaving me in private with their kids. Even though I was not a mother at the time, some moms also saw the interview as an opportunity to give me advice "for the future."

I believe that my racial identity, in particular my racial ambiguity, was helpful overall, though at times it seemed to make mothers uncomfortable. I am neither white nor clearly ethnically identifiable (although my name certainly hints at my ethnic origins). Because most moms knew that I didn't share their racial/ethnic backgrounds, they couldn't take for granted that I'd understand their diets. This motivated them to explain things to me clearly and in great detail. They discussed the role of particular dishes in cultural traditions and celebrations, and they laid out for me the ingredients in family recipes. But sometimes, I could tell that my identity sowed discomfort in families, and I wondered how that might have altered their accounts. I interviewed one white mom who repeatedly told me over the course of an hour how much she enjoyed "ethnic food." Finally, after fifty minutes, she asked what my "specific ethnicity" was, at which point she began explaining how much she loved Indian food. She listed some Indian restaurants in the area and shared her favorite dishes, perhaps in an effort to prove her cultural competence to me. Ultimately, while I tried to meet families where they were and be as open as possible, I had to come to terms with the fact that my appearance and presence shaped their accounts in ways beyond my control.

I recorded every conversation so that I could be present and fully attentive during interviews. This left me with hundreds of hours of interviews to listen to and transcribe.[5] But there was more to capturing interviews than just relistening and rereading dialogue. Immediately after every interview, I spent hours sitting on the stool at my kitchen counter replaying each recording and writing up field notes. These notes were filled with detailed descriptions of what I had observed: people's facial expressions and clothing, their interactions with each other, the smell of their apartments, the comfort or tension that permeated the conversation.

As I wrote down the facts, I also put into words what I was learning and how my own understanding of families' diets was evolving. What had that interview taught me? How had this interview aligned with or diverged from others? Writing field notes was how I made sense of my data. By the time I sat down in 2016 to formally analyze thousands of pages of interview transcripts, this process had already given me a sense of what these analyses might uncover.

Beyond families' stories, interviews offered countless opportunities to observe their diets in action. Mothers whom I met in cafés often bought breakfast and lunch, and teens showed up to interviews with snacks in hand. More than a few times, I stepped into families' living rooms to find a smorgasbord of appetizers laid out in anticipation of my arrival. Some made me lunch; others asked if I wanted to look through their fridges. I sampled samosas and collard greens, quesadillas and cheesecake.

These relatively brief observations showed me that more extensive, sustained observations were key to unpacking families' food choices. These would also showcase how food fit within the contours of family life. But to my knowledge, no one had collected these kinds of data yet. So I decided to ask four families I'd interviewed if I could observe them.

All four met my request with a subtle blend of curiosity and confusion. Nyah, Dana, Renata, and Julie all wanted to know what exactly I'd be observing, whether they should act normal or plan something special for my visits, and if it would be "weird." I told them the truth—that I was interested in everything about their lives and that I absolutely did not want them to make special plans for my visits. They should simply live their lives as normal, whether that meant preparing a four-course meal or watching *So You Think You Can Dance* while baking a frozen lasagna.

"Are you sure you want to study *us?*" Dana squinted at me during my first home visit. It was a Tuesday evening, and we were sitting on her living-room couch watching Paige entertain us with somersault after somersault.

"Absolutely," I assured her. Then, smiling, I motioned to Paige, who had somersaulted herself into a fit of laughter. "I wouldn't want to miss this."

"Okay!" Dana laughed and looked at me quizzically. "If you say so."

Ultimately, all four families opened their doors to me. I started observing them during different hours of the day, on different days of the week, and at different places. Food was front and center during mealtimes and trips to the supermarket, but I also came to appreciate food's omnipresence in daily life. Food snuck its way into countless moments, big and small: during trips to the mall and in the car, at graduation parties and after dance recitals. Because food was everywhere, I too tried to be everywhere. The more time I spent with each family, the more hospitality they showed me, welcoming me into their lives in unexpected ways. I began by asking to tag along to different outings, but soon I found myself getting invited to birthday parties, holiday celebrations, and cheerleading competitions, and to meet extended family and friends.

While observing, I thought about what to do with myself. How should I behave? How could I ensure that I was neither a burden nor an unintentional influence on families' behaviors? Sociologists have long asked questions like these, debating the researcher's role in ethnographic observations. There are no simple answers. Some scholars propose that the ethnographer should be an unobtrusive observer, while others advocate for becoming a full-fledged participant in people's lives.

My approach fell somewhere between these two poles but edged toward observation over participation. Most of the time, I tried to settle into the background and watch events unfold naturally. The first day I observed a family was generally a bit awkward. But that soon changed, and assuming a fly-on-the-wall approach helped me become a taken-for-granted fixture in families' lives. Parents and kids fought, argued, played, gossiped, and went about their daily lives with little regard for my presence.

When it wasn't obvious how to act, I tried to read the moment. Most of the time, this led me to take a more hands-off approach. I avoided inserting myself physically or verbally into a situation. But moments sometimes arose when remaining peripheral or detached felt either inappropriate or damaging to the relationships I was building. It's one thing to remain silent when no one asks your opinion; it's another to actively avoid answering questions or decline an invitation. These refusals may come from a place of not wanting to unduly influence a situation, but they come at a cost. On top of simply being rude, not engaging can destroy hard-earned trust and rapport and thus compromise an ethnographer's ability to continue conducting research.

So when families tried to include me, I let myself be included. I boiled rice, stirred pasta sauce, discussed the news, and weighed in on prom dresses. I shared parts of my life with families too, including childhood memories, weekend plans, favorite dishes, and my plan to write a book. Sometimes I assumed the role of a casual but inquisitive interviewer, asking questions to understand what was happening around me. One Wednesday I accompanied Renata to her church's service, which took place in an auditorium that could easily hold two thousand people. I noticed ten minutes in that she was treating our visit like a guided tour, introducing me to the pastor and showing me where the youth service was held. I mirrored her approach, asking questions along the way. "When did you start coming here?" I inquired as we took our seats and waited for the service to begin. A Christian rock band—with José on the drums—kicked off the service, and lyrics flashed across a sprawling screen. I joined Renata in singing along. Another afternoon we sat on the couch eating Papa John's and watching the TV show *The Voice*.

"Who are you rooting for?" I asked her, biting into my cheese pizza. Through it all, I strove to be someone that families enjoyed having around. I tried to be kind and a good listener and to always engage with humility.

I wrote down detailed notes while observing families, but, as with interviews, I also spent hours after each observation session typing up field notes. Since my goal was to understand families' lives—and how food fit into those lives—I made note of anything I saw happen at home, from family feuds to a broken washing machine. I worked tirelessly to link what I saw happening in their lives with what I observed was happening with their diets.[6]

I decided to embed myself within families to closely examine and seek to understand the textures of their lives. But I was keenly attuned to the dynamics of power and privilege inherent in these kinds of researcher-respondent relationships.

This meant that I worried constantly about doing right by families. This concern in part drove me to financially compensate families for interviews and observations. Allowing me to observe them would require some effort on their end—coordinating with me, working out any necessary logistics, letting me steal a pizza bagel or two—and I was deeply uncomfortable with a dynamic of me as researcher "taking" without offering anything in return. All four moms were interested in the money, but, unsurprisingly, it meant much more to Nyah and Dana.

Still, I discovered that families weren't just financially motivated to participate. They shared personal motives as well. The fact that I took a genuine interest in their lives meant something to the moms I spent time with. While it is neither my intention nor a broadcasted "benefit," participating in the research offered them a rare opportunity to be the center of attention and the recognized experts on their own lives. In a small way, moms became the heroes of a story I was documenting.

That said, it was always clear to me that I was documenting these stories as an outsider. I knew that no matter how well I came to know any one family, I would never personally—in any way, shape, or form—experience their lives as they did. I would not weather the same losses, confront the same challenges, or face the same hardships. Similarly, I would not mark the same milestones or revel in the same victories. Each evening, I would retreat to the studio apartment that I rented as a graduate student, to the academic seminars where I read books and wrote papers, and to an impeccably manicured college campus that felt starkly disconnected from the world I observed. While I was there *with* families, I never tried to become *of* them.

And yet, knowing full well the impossibility of walking a mile in a family's shoes, I was fortunate that they granted me the chance to briefly walk alongside them. They helped me discover the most essential tool of social science: withholding judgment. Withholding judgment isn't the same thing as objectivity. Social scientific research, like any human enterprise, can never be objective. When I stepped into families' homes, I always brought who I was, what I looked like, and what I'd experienced with me. My identities and histories shaped all aspects of my study. Objectivity is beyond my control.

But a concerted effort to refrain from judgment lies well within it.

As much as possible, I refrained. Of course, as a human being, I did not always find this easy or achievable. Some moments tested my limits. But whenever I fell off the horse, I carefully climbed back on again. I worked to watch families carefully. I listened closely. I questioned my reactions. I wrestled with my confusions. I called out my biases. I shifted my paradigms. I repeatedly strove to replace feelings of judgment with ones of sincere curiosity. And in doing so, I noticed two things. First, the more families sensed that I was not judging them, the more readily they allowed me to see behind the curtain. Second, the more I refrained from judgment, the wider my mind opened and the more deeply I came to appreciate the fuller context and circumstances of families' lives. Choices that may have seemed strange from the outside revealed themselves to me as perfectly reasonable and rational.

A keener ability to see the rational in what was generally deemed irrational translated into a more grounded, empathetic, and responsive research process. This process infused my interactions and relationships with families. It also—I sincerely hope—shaped how I wrote this book for the better.

I remember one evening when I accompanied Dana to Walmart to get Madison and Paige new clothes and snacks for the week. The trip had been challenging, as the girls had bombarded Dana with endless requests. Could she get them Fruity Pebbles, a new bike helmet, a two-piece swimsuit? Dana couldn't really afford any of those things, at least not on that day. The last light of dusk faded as we pulled into the driveway after the exhausting outing. Her foot on the brake, Dana let the girls out. She and I sat alone in the front seats. Dana put the car in park before dropping her head into her hands. And there, completely overwhelmed and overtired, she started to cry. It was a soft cry, but unmistakably raw and vulnerable.

With no tissue to offer, I offered, instead, my ear. Gingerly placing my hand on her shoulder, I listened quietly as she told me all about the struggles with family and friends that kept her up at night. Her sister's cancer diagnosis. Her ex-husband's drug problem. The electricity bill. The cost of gymnastics camp. Dana shared, and I listened like I knew what she was talking about, because by that point, I did. Moments like this deepened my understanding of everything moms like Dana were going through. They helped me connect the dots between the countless moving parts of families' lives and the food that graced their plates. And these moments also reminded me that if there was ever a question—if I ever had to choose—I would always decide to be a human first and a researcher second.

I'm often asked how this research changed me. Especially now, as a mother, how did spending so much time studying kids' diets affect how I approach my daughter's? People generally assume that the research made me care more about what I feed her. How could spending that much time researching kids' diets *not* make someone obsessed with her own child's intake?

In fact, the research had the opposite effect on me.

It's not that I don't want Veda to eat nutritiously. Like most moms, I do. Also like most moms, my child's health and well-being are of the utmost importance to me. But this research solidified a truth I'd known for decades, a truth that had lodged itself beneath my rib cage the first day I'd interacted with the foster-care system at nine years old. That truth is that I am profoundly lucky. This luck is what set me on one trajectory and my foster siblings on another. Now, as a mom, this same luck affords me luxuries in this country—like stable housing and a livable wage—that shape how I feed my daughter.

I cannot, after being touched by so many moms' stories and struggles, take these luxuries for granted. I am privileged to be able to afford not only healthy food but also many other things I wish to give my daughter. Society has not backed me into a situation where I have to use food to buffer my child against hardship. I do not need to sacrifice my satiation for hers, and I have the means to take shortcuts when necessary, or even convenient, to secure the nutritious food I want. I always knew these were luxuries, but my research helped me *feel* it. I can temper any of my worries that sprout up about Veda eating a bowl of sugary cereal or drinking a can of soda with the knowledge that, in this country, these luxuries stack the deck in my favor as a mom and in hers as my daughter.

The research also made me angrier. Motherhood is hard, but there are so many ways that America makes it an untenable struggle, whether through an inadequate federal safety net, a consistent prioritization of corporate interests over families' health, an insidious rhetoric of personal (often maternal) over social responsibility, or a general devaluation of all things deemed "women's work," feeding included. Seeing moms' struggles made me extremely wary and resentful of intensive-mothering standards. In a country that offers such limited support to families, I resented the onslaught of expectations and judgment that seemed to go hand in hand with motherhood. Why should moms always be primary caregivers, multitaskers, and overinformed self-sacrificers? I felt furious for the moms I met. And as a mother myself, I didn't want to feel like I was constantly failing—like I was never enough.

And yet, that *is* how I sometimes feel. There are moments when, as a mother, I feel inadequate, less-than, selfish. More often than I'd like to admit, a deep desire bubbles up in me to prove my commitment and devotion to my daughter. I want to show beyond a doubt to her, myself, and others how "good" I am.

In those moments, I call the moms from this research to the front of my mind. I think of the countless mothers I met who inspired me with their perseverance and grit, imagination, and resourcefulness. They remind me that, like them and despite how it can feel, I *am* good. We all are. Me, Nyah, Dana, Renata, Julie, Ximena, Janae, Sonali. We are all good moms. We love and nourish our children however we can. We make it work, whatever the circumstances. There is no question that our kids are our world. But as moms, we deserve to live in a society built of infinitely more empathy, appreciation, and support.

Acknowledgments

To the families who opened your doors to me: thank you for your generosity and candor, and for granting me the privilege of hearing your stories. Nyah, Dana, Renata, and Julie—you are the heart and soul of this book, and I feel immensely fortunate to know each of you. I only hope that, through these pages, I have done justice to your struggles, ingenuity, and courage.

My literary agent, Jessica Papin, catapulted my dream of becoming an author into a reality. She was instrumental at every turn, and I'm grateful for her unwavering belief in this work and in me as a writer. "This is going to be an important book, Priya!" she once e-mailed me when I had hit a low point in the writing process. Her optimism and encouragement were exactly what I needed to keep my head down and continue putting words to the page. This book is infinitely better because it had her as its fiercest advocate.

During my first conversation with my editor, Marisa Vigilante, it quickly became clear to me that her grasp of the book's potential and contribution far exceeded my own. Thank you, Marisa, for always being able to step back and share the bigger picture with me, for your graceful, incisive editing, and for simply getting it. Working with you has been an incredible privilege. To the rest of the team at Little, Brown Spark and Hachette—Tracy Behar, Ian Straus, Fanta Diallo, Jayne Yaffe Kemp, Carolyn Levin, Jessica Chun, Juliana Horbachevsky, and

Stephanie Reddaway—I appreciate all of the hard work you devoted to this book and the way you guided me as a first-time author. Thank you to Tracy Roe for her expert copyediting and attention to detail, and to Deborah Jacobs for her meticulous proofreading.

This book grew out of research I conducted as a doctoral student at Stanford University. I'm grateful for my colleagues and mentors within the Department of Sociology who guided me and helped shape me as a scholar. My dissertation adviser, Tomás Jiménez, opened my eyes early on to the craft of qualitative methods and the art of data-driven storytelling. Tomás advocated tirelessly for this project and saw it through to the end, reading an early draft of the manuscript and offering astute feedback that strengthened its sociological contributions. Throughout the research, Doug McAdam and Michelle Jackson provided pivotal support and keen insights; their ongoing encouragement helped me keep putting one foot in front of the other. Countless faculty and doctoral students within the department's Gender and Social Psychology; Migration, Ethnicity, Race and Nation; Qualitative Methods; and Inequality workshops offered helpful feedback, suggestions, and advice through the years that sculpted the research at the heart of the book.

At the Stanford Center on Poverty and Inequality, David Grusky, Kathryn Edin, and Charles Varner helped deepen my understanding of the causes and contours of poverty and inequality in America while granting me key opportunities to expand my methodological expertise. My time as a Graduate Dissertation Fellow at the Clayman Institute for Gender Research changed me personally and professionally. My colleagues and mentors at the institute—including Shelley Correll, Alison Dahl Crossley, Lori Nishiura Mackenzie, Caroline Simard, Sara Jordan-Bloch, Aliya Rao, Alison Wynn, Melissa Abad, Wendy Skidmore, and Kristine Kilanski—were instrumental in tightening and adding nuance to my analysis of food and gender inequality within families. Before I had the confidence to trust my own ideas and sociological intuition, Marianne Cooper carried that confidence for me; she was the first person to believe that this project mattered and that I was the right person to execute it. Her conviction gave me the guts to take a requisite leap of faith.

I was immensely fortunate to receive a number of grants and fellowships that gave me the time and funding necessary to pursue this research during my doctoral studies. I am grateful to Stanford University's Office of the Vice Provost for Graduate Education and Department of Sociology, Haas Center for Public Service, McCoy Family Center for Ethics in Society, Center on Philanthropy and Civil Society, Clayman Institute for Gender Research, and Center on Poverty and Inequality for their critical financial support and for significantly enriching my worldview.

I'm extremely grateful to my research assistants who aided me through all stages of the work. During the writing process, Caroline Aung helped me present the bigger picture by digging up important information about families, inequality, and food policy in America. Caroline additionally carefully read various chapters and offered pointed insights to improve their tone and substance. I'm thankful to the many transcribers who turned hundreds of hours of audio recordings of interviews into written transcripts that I could pore over for analysis—thank you to Arianna Wassman, Apoorva Handigol, Catherine Zaw, Corinna Brendel, Laura Figueroa, Maria Deloso, Michaela Elias, Elen Mendoza, Minjia Zhong, Sarah McCurdy, Sarah Roberts, Sarah Techavarutama, and Victor Verdejo.

It was a privilege to write this book as a postdoctoral fellow at the Stanford School of Medicine, where I was generously funded by a National Institutes of Health T32 training grant. I am grateful to Christopher Gardner, Jodi Prochaska, and Tom Robinson at the Stanford Prevention Research Center for their support. In particular, thank you to Christopher for his hands-on, relentlessly positive mentorship and for providing thoughtful, heartening comments on an early draft. I wrote much of this book in the midst of a pandemic without childcare; Christopher ensured I had the time, space, and moral support to get the job done. Eventually, I was able to keep writing with the caregiving support of Francineia Peres. Thank you, Fran, for providing my daughter with abundant love, attention, and care, thereby allowing me to focus on bringing this book to life. Revising this book took just about as long as writing it did. I'm also thankful to my colleagues at the Center for Health Outcomes and Population Equity at Huntsman Cancer Institute as well as the Department of Family and Consumer Studies at the University of Utah for their support as I worked my way through revisions.

When I wanted to author a trade book but knew neither where nor how to begin, I turned to Thomas Hayden. Tom took me under his wing, mentored me through countless book-proposal drafts, and remained a devoted advocate through the entire process. Thank you, Tom, for being in my corner; I can confidently say that this book would not exist without you. Thank you also to Lauren Oakes for providing an inspiring model of engaged, public-facing scholarship that excited and motivated me through all stages of this process.

I am indebted to my dear friends who generously read full drafts of this book and provided focused line edits, multipage editorial write-ups, and multi-hour phone calls to discuss and troubleshoot. Aditi Mehta, Neel Lalchandani, Eric Xiyu Li, Devon Magliozzi, and Laura O'Donohue—I can never thank you enough for all the time you spent helping me. Your kind and constructive insights fundamentally shaped the end product. When I found myself with just two weeks left to finish my manuscript, Jennifer Wang performed a feat of magic and big friendship by reading and providing careful, detailed comments on the entire book in a remarkably short period of time. Thank you, Jen, for your selflessness, for the e-mail you sent me at 4:09 a.m., and for your enduring friendship.

I am indebted to my close friends, fellow sociologists, and feminist-book-club members Christianne Corbett, Catherine Sirois, Chloe Grace Hart, and Madeline Young. Thank you for being endless wells of inspiration and encouragement, not to mention faithful readers whose brilliance strengthened the book's arguments and sociological foci. Alissa Dos Santos and Bethany Nichols, from whom I never stop learning, provided wise suggestions on various chapters that bolstered my voice and regrounded me in the narrative. Other collaborators, colleagues, and friends across Stanford and sociology were ongoing sources of emotional and intellectual support through the years; my sincerest thank-you to Swethaa Ballakrishnen, Natalie Jabbar, Christof Brandtner, Caitlin Daniel, Lisa Hummel, Molly King, Adam Horowitz, Sandra Nakagawa, Juan Pedroza, Nicole Ardoin, and Rachel Wright.

For their friendship, I am eternally grateful to Carolyn Donohue, Caroline Lopez, Cristina Pappas, Michelle Alden, Jill Fay, Lindley Mease, David Wei, Holly Harridan, Maja Falcon, Whitney Vallabhaneni, Michele Lanpher Patel, Elizabeth Talbert, Justin Kreindler, Shadie Parivar, and Joel Weitzman. Thank you to Lizzy Kreindler for her kind spirit, humor, and sisterhood. The truth is that so much of what I've accomplished in my life is because I've had such a generous, compassionate, and caring friend to bring the wind to my sails when I've needed it most.

I have had the immense fortune to stand upon the shoulders of my family. I thank my mom and dad for their steady encouragement, boundless support, and measured optimism and for raising me with the courage to chart my own path. Thank you to my brothers and greatest teachers, Vikram and Josh. Connie, Ethan, Owen, Mama, Bapa, Bubu Bhai, Bhabhi, Anya, Nivan, Sonu, Alyssa, Kim, Steph — thank you for steadfastly believing in me and for offering me a soft place to land.

To Veda, who came into my life when I was in the middle of writing this book, whom I nursed and rocked and bathed and clutched in the moments I was not typing these pages: Before you arrived, I worried about whether I could write a book (something I'd never done before) while caring for a newborn (another thing I'd never done before). Now I know the truth—that I could not have done it without you. Your sincerity and spirit gave me a reason to write, and you helped me see with new eyes and feel with a freer heart. We, this book and I, are better because of you.

Lastly, to Ansu—you once told me that my dreams were your dreams; my aspirations, your aspirations; my happiness, your happiness. Never—not once—have I doubted this. Thank you for your brilliance and bigheartedness. Through it all, you have stood beside me, your fingers interlaced with mine. I am grateful every day for your unwavering belief in me and for how, in my moments of doubt, you boldly reflect my dreams back to me.

Notes

Preface

1. With their permission, I have used the real names of my brother and my spouse. To accurately and precisely reconstruct our conversations and experiences, I corroborated my own memories, journal entries, documents, and records with theirs.

2. Despite BMI's imprecision and limitations, it continues to be used for a few reasons. First, it's not always inaccurate; BMI correctly categorizes people as having excess body fat more than 80 percent of the time. But second, and perhaps more important, there are currently few acceptable alternatives. While there are certainly more precise measures of body fat (for instance, MRI scans), these are often expensive and labor-intensive and therefore difficult to use across health-care settings. Many scientists and clinicians agree that BMI is useful when examining a population over time but limited at the individual level; BMI measurements are most valuable as an initial screening tool and to identify individuals who may be at risk for certain conditions or diseases. For more about the merits and drawbacks of BMI, see "Measuring Obesity," Harvard T. H. Chan School of Public Health, January 2021, https://www.hsph.harvard.edu/obesity-prevention-source/obesity-definition/how-to-measure-body-fatness/, and Carla Kemp, "Merits, Drawbacks of BMI Measurement to Be Debated," *American Academy of Pediatrics News*, September 15, 2017.

Chapter 1: Diverging Destinies

1. Emphasis is mine. For a discussion of radical empathy, see Isabel Wilkerson, *Caste: The Origins of Our Discontents* (New York: Penguin, 2020).

2. Overall, nutritionists agree that healthy diets consist of more plant-based, whole foods and fewer processed foods and foods with added sugar. In 2015, the food-education nonprofit Oldways hosted a conference during which they asked twenty-one nutrition scientists of all beliefs and backgrounds to align on a definition of *healthy eating*. The group was

chaired by nutrition professors David Katz and Walter Willett and included Mediterranean diet researcher Miguel Martínez-González, Paleo diet founder S. Boyd Eaton, and vegan-diet promoter Neal Barnard. After two days of debate, the scientists came to eleven points of consensus, including a definition of a healthy diet that broadly aligned with the food-based recommendations of the 2015 *DGA*. They also agreed with the *DGA* that a focus on foods—rather than just fats, carbs, and protein in isolation—was preferable. See Caroline Praderio, "9 Things the World's Top Nutrition Experts All Agree On," *Prevention* (December 9, 2015).

Nutritionists Tim Spector and Christopher Gardner reflected on the 2018 Food for Thought nutrition meeting, which was convened by the *British Medical Journal* and Swiss Re. The meeting brought together scientists, health practitioners, and journalists to discuss controversies and consensus in nutrition and health. Spector and Gardner write that during those discussions, there was broad consensus that healthy diets are rich in fiber, vegetables, and fruits and low in sugar and ultra-processed foods. They note, however, that there was less consensus on other issues, particularly dietary advice for patients with diabetes, the benefits of keto diets, and the role of meat, saturated fats, and salt restriction. See Tim Spector and Christopher Gardner, "Challenges and Opportunities for Better Nutrition Science," *British Medical Journal* 369 (June 2020): m2470.

In his 2020 American Heart Association talk entitled "Better Nutrition Studies," Christopher Gardner also notes that nutrition studies are uniquely complex and that there is general agreement that the basis of a good fundamental diet includes more vegetables and whole foods and less added sugar, refined grains, and processed foods. See Alexander C. Razavi et al., "EPI/Lifestyle Scientific Sessions: 2020 Meeting Highlights," *Journal of the American Heart Association* 9 (June 2020): e017252.

3. U.S. Department of Health and Human Services and U.S. Department of Agriculture, *2020–2025 Dietary Guidelines for Americans,* 9th edition, December 2020, https://health.gov/our-work/food-nutrition/current-dietary-guidelines.

4. Researchers use different scales to measure the quality of people's diets. These scales typically measure the amount of fruits and vegetables, whole grains, fish and shellfish, sugar-sweetened beverages, nuts, seeds, legumes, and processed meat people are eating. For some of these foods, like fruits and vegetables, higher intake means a higher score, while it's the opposite for others, like sugar-sweetened beverages. Researchers add up the individual food group scores to get a total score of diet quality for each person. To be sure, these metrics and their associated methods are imperfect. To collect data on people's diets, interviewers generally call people on the phone and ask them to recall what they have eaten, in fine detail, over the past twenty-four hours. They use strategies to help people remember and report their consumption accurately, but since these data

are based on people's own recollections and reporting, they are subject to interviewees' memory lapses and misinterpretations. Even though these scales vary in their specifics and are imperfect, most national studies using them yield largely the same findings about overall American dietary intake.

5. M. M. Wilson, J. Reedy, and S. M. Krebs-Smith, "American Diet Quality: Where It Is, Where It Is Heading, and What It Could Be," *Journal of the Academy of Nutrition and Dietetics* 116 (February 2016): 302–10.

6. "Poor Nutrition," National Center for Chronic Disease Prevention and Health Promotion, April 14, 2020, www.cdc.gov/chronicdisease/resources /publications/factsheets/nutrition.htm. The overconsumption of calories is in part evidenced by the fact that two-thirds of all adults in the United States are either overweight or obese. This is double the rate of obesity from thirty years ago. These trends hold for kids too; over the last thirty years, obesity rates have tripled among children and quadrupled among adolescents. Nearly one-third of children are now obese or overweight. See Cheryl Fryar et al., "Prevalence of Overweight, Obesity, and Extreme Obesity Among Adults: United States, 1960–1962 Through 2011–2012," National Center for Health Statistics, November 6, 2015, www.cdc.gov /nchs/data/hestat/obesity_adult_11_12/obesity_adult_11_12.htm.

7. Junxiu Liu et al., "Trends in Diet Quality Among Youth in the United States, 1999–2016," *Journal of the American Medical Association* 323, no. 12 (March 24, 2020): 1161–74, https://jamanetwork.com/journals/jama /fullarticle/2763291.

8. F. F. Zhang et al., "Trends and Disparities in Diet Quality Among US Adults by Supplemental Nutrition Assistance Program Participation Status," *JAMA Network Open* 1 (2018): e180237; D. D. Wang et al., "Trends in Dietary Quality Among Adults in the United States, 1999 Through 2010," *JAMA Internal Medicine* 174 (2014): 1587–95; Y. Wang and X. Chen, "How Much of Racial/Ethnic Disparities in Dietary Intakes, Exercise, and Weight Status Can Be Explained by Nutrition- and Health-Related Psychosocial Factors and Socioeconomic Status Among US Adults?," *Journal of the American Dietetic Association* 111 (2011): 1904–11.

9. Liu et al., "Trends in Diet Quality Among Youth"; A. D. Guerrero and P. J. Chung, "Racial and Ethnic Disparities in Dietary Intake Among California Children," *Journal of the Academy of Nutrition and Dietetics* 116, no. 3 (2016): 439–48.

10. US Burden of Disease Collaborators, "The State of US Health, 1990–2016," *Journal of the American Medical Association* 319, no. 14 (April 2018): 1444–72, https://jamanetwork.com/journals/jama/fullarticle/2678018.

11. Type 2 diabetes illustrates these disparities, as it disproportionately affects low-income communities and those of color. Approximately 13 percent of adults without a high-school education have diagnosed diabetes, compared to 9.7 percent of those with a high-school education and 7.5 percent of those with more than a high-school education. Counties with the greatest rates of poverty have the highest rates of diabetes. Similarly, the risk of developing type 2 is 77 percent higher for

Black people and 66 percent higher for Hispanic people than it is for white individuals. Asian-Americans, Native Hawaiians, and Pacific Islanders have the highest rates and twice the risk of developing diabetes than the general population. Overall, 12.5 percent of Hispanic and 11.7 percent of Black people have type 2 diabetes, compared to 7.5 percent of white people. See *National Diabetes Statistics Report 2020: Estimates of Diabetes and Its Burden in the United States,* Centers for Disease Control and Prevention (2020): 1–32, and James A. Levine, "Poverty and Obesity in the U.S.," *Diabetes* 60, no. 11 (November 2011): 2667–68.

12. For more information on economic inequality in the U.S., see Drew DeSilver, "U.S. Income Inequality, on Rise for Decades, Is Now Highest Since 1928," Pew Research Center, December 5, 2013; Elise Gould, "Decades of Rising Economic Inequality in the U.S.: Testimony Before the U.S. House of Representatives Ways and Means Committee," Economic Policy Institute, March 27, 2019; Isabel V. Sawhill and Christopher Pulliam, "Six Facts About Wealth in the United States," Brookings Institution, June 28, 2019; Estelle Sommeiller and Mark Price, "The New Gilded Age: Income Inequality in the US by State, Metropolitan Area, and County," Economic Policy Institute, July 19, 2018; Robert Reich, *Saving Capitalism: For the Many, Not the Few* (New York: Penguin, 2015).

   The Gini coefficient is also a common and intuitive metric. Its value can fall between 0 and 1, with the former indicating perfect equality (where everyone has the same income) and the latter perfect inequality (where one person has all the income, and everyone else no income). America's Gini coefficient has been rising for the past five decades and is higher than that of social-welfare states with stronger safety nets such as Sweden and France. For more information, see Gloria Guzman, "New Data Show Income Increased in 14 States and 10 of the Largest Metros," United States Census Bureau, September 26, 2019, https://www.census.gov/library/stories/2019/09/us-median-household-income-up-in-2018-from-2017.html.

13. For more on the durability and intergenerational transfer of inequality, see Richard V. Reeves and Katherine Guyot, "Fewer Americans Are Making More than Their Parents Did—Especially If They Grew Up in the Middle Class," Brookings Institution, October 12, 2018; Raj Chetty et al., "The Fading American Dream: Trends in Absolute Income Mobility Since 1940," *Science* 356, no. 6336 (2017): 398–406.

   Intersecting economic and racial inequalities coalesce to produce "diverging destinies" for kids. Those born into privilege are more likely to be raised in an environment of financial security and family and housing stability; those born into less privileged families are more likely to grow up with greater precariousness in these dimensions. Black, brown, and low-income children face major barriers to their health, including inadequate health-care access, greater exposure to environmental pollutants and contaminants, and more experiences of detrimental toxic stress. As a result, they have comparatively higher rates of disease, including obesity, type 2 diabetes, and asthma, along with learning disabilities and poor oral health. Altogether, children from marginalized communities face what's called a concentration of disadvantage, preventing them from accessing opportunities to get ahead. For more on families, poverty, and inequality in America, see Kathryn Edin and H. Luke Shaefer, *$2.00 a Day: Living on Almost Nothing in America* (New York: Mariner, 2016); Barbara Ehrenreich, *Nickel and Dimed: On (Not) Getting By in America* (New York: Henry Holt, 2011); P. J. Smock and C. R. Schwartz, "The Demography of Families: A Review of Patterns and Change," *Journal of Marriage and Family* 82, no. 1 (2020): 9–34; "Child Poverty," National Center for Children in Poverty, Bank Street Graduate School of Education, 2019; Julie E. Artis, "Maternal Cohabitation and Child Well-Being Among Kindergarten Children," *Journal of Marriage and Family* 69, no. 1 (January 2007): 222–36; Paula Fomby and Andrew J. Cherlin, "Family Instability and Child Well-Being," *American Sociological Review* 72, no. 2 (2007): 181–204; S. McLanahan and W. Jacobson, "Diverging Destinies Revisited," in *Families in an Era of Increasing Inequality: Diverging Destinies*, ed. P. R. Amato et al. (Basel, Switzerland: Springer, 2015), 3–23; Marianne Cooper and Allison Pugh, "Families Across the Income Spectrum: A Decade in Review," *Journal of Marriage and Family* 82, no. 1 (February 2020): 272–99.

14. America trails other Western industrialized nations in the reach of its social safety net, with many European welfare states better at redistributing income among their citizens on a large scale, providing social programs that reach a wide share of citizens, and offering more progressive tax systems. In contrast, the U.S. government has historically refrained from assuming responsibility for residents' well-being. For more information on the lack of affordable childcare and paid family leave, see Swapna Venugopal Ramaswamy et al., "America's Parents Want Paid Family Leave and Affordable Child Care. Why Can't They Get It?," *USA Today*, December 3, 2019, and Alberto Alesina et al., "Why Doesn't the United States Have a European-Style Welfare State?," *Brookings Papers on Economic Activity* 2 (2001): 187–272.

15. Christine Percheski and Christina Gibson-Davis, "A Penny on the Dollar: Racial Inequalities in Wealth Among Households with Children," *Socius* (June 2020).

16. For more about racial inequalities and COVID-19, see M. Chowkwanyun and A. L. Reed, "Racial Health Disparities and Covid-19—Caution and Context," *New England Journal of Medicine* 383, no. 3 (2020): 201–203, and Rashawn Ray, "Why Are Blacks Dying at Higher Rates from COVID-19?," Brookings Institution, April 9, 2020. For more on the links between nutrition and COVID-19, see M. J. Belanger et al., "COVID-19 and Disparities in Nutrition and Obesity," *New England Journal of Medicine* (July 2020).

17. For a deeper, riveting dive into the drawbacks and constraints of the foster-care system, see Larissa MacFarquhar, "When Should a Child Be Taken from His Parents?," *New Yorker*, July 31, 2017.

Chapter 2: Families in an Age of Inequality

1. D. D. Wang et al., "Trends in Dietary Quality Among Adults in the United States, 1999 Through 2010," *JAMA Internal Medicine* 174, no. 10 (2014): 1587–95, doi:10.1001/jamainternmed.2014.3422.

2. Monetary values are adjusted to pertain to a family of four in 2018 dollars. See Sarah Bohn and Tess Thorman, "Just the Facts: Income Inequality in California," Public Policy Institute of California, January 2020.

3. Katherine Schaeffer, "Among U.S. Couples, Women Do More Cooking and Grocery Shopping than Men," Pew Research Center, September 24, 2019.

4. Dana Williams's biological mother was white and her biological father was Puerto Rican. Dana was raised by two white parents and was white-passing. Both of her daughters' fathers were white, and her daughters were also white-passing.

5. Matthew Desmond, *Evicted: Profit and Poverty in the American City* (New York: Crown, 2016).

6. For more on weathering, see Arline T. Geronimus, "The Weathering Hypothesis and the Health of African-American Women and Infants: Evidence and Speculations," *Ethnicity and Disease* 2, no. 3 (1992): 207–21; Arline T. Geronimus, "Black/White Differences in the Relationship of Maternal Age to Birthweight: A Population-Based Test of the Weathering Hypothesis," *Social Science and Medicine* 42, no. 4 (1996): 589–97; Arline T. Geronimus, "'Weathering' and Age-Patterns of Allostatic Load Scores Among Blacks and Whites in the United States," *American Journal of Public Health* (2006): 826–33; Gene Demby, "Making the Case That Discrimination Is Bad for Your Health," *Code Switch* (podcast), NPR, January 14, 2018.

Chapter 3: Feeding Kids

1. Most moms leveraged a mainstream healthy-eating discourse, a way of thinking and speaking about food that is increasingly popular and widespread in America today. This discourse's pervasiveness illustrates how most people across society believe in the importance of healthy eating and share broadly similar understandings of what is healthy and what is unhealthy. For more information on the mainstream healthy-eating discourse, see Brenda Beagan et al., *Acquired Tastes: Why Families Eat the Way They Do* (Vancouver, Canada: UBC Press, 2017).

2. One reason for my surprise was that I had heard so many times before that poor parents were not knowledgeable about healthy eating. How many articles and tweets had I come across that implied that poor people were ignorant about food? That they didn't know that a Big Mac and fries weren't healthy? That they didn't know what an eggplant or kiwi was? While there is some research showing that poor parents may have lower knowledge of specific nutrient groups, other research suggests that they are just as knowledgeable about food groups and healthy and unhealthy products. See P. A. Cluss et al., "Nutrition Knowledge of Low-Income

Parents of Obese Children," *Translational Behavioral Medicine* 3, no. 2 (2013): 218–25.

3. For more information about targeted food and beverage marketing to youth of color, see Jennifer Harris and Willie Frazier III, "Increasing Disparities in Unhealthy Food Advertising Targeted to Hispanic and Black Youth," Rudd Center for Food Policy and Obesity (2019). The food industry also spent twenty-eight billion dollars in lobbying politicians at the federal level. See "Industry Profile: Food and Beverage Lobbying, 2019," OpenSecrets.org, 2020, and "Food and Beverages," Statista.com, 2020.

4. These are just examples of what we can see. Other, largely invisible aspects of the food environment also push us toward processed foods. Agricultural policies shape how foods are grown on farms in what quantities, which foods appear in our supermarkets, and what they cost. Countless federal, state, and local efforts exist to collaborate and collude with (and sometimes regulate) the food and beverage industries, affecting everything from food labels to brand marketing to which foods make it into school vending machines, cafeterias, and fundraisers. See "Why We Overeat: The Toxic Food Environment and Obesity," Harvard T. H. Chan School of Public Health, September 13, 2013, https://the forum.sph.harvard.edu/events/why-we-overeat/.

5. There are several important causes of the unhealthy food environment. Since the deregulation of the food and beverage industry in the 1980s, this environment has become increasingly toxic. It starts on farms, where, beginning in the 1970s, the federal government started subsidizing certain crops to support rural communities and manage hunger by assuring that consumers had a plentiful supply of food at reasonable prices. Today, the U.S. government still spends billions of dollars every year to provide subsidies to farmers. The vast majority of federal agricultural subsidies finances the production of corn, soybeans, wheat, rice, sorghum, dairy, and livestock. Many of these products are converted into refined grains, high-fat and high-sodium processed foods, and high-calorie juices and soft drinks. These subsidies help keep the prices of those products down. Not surprisingly, these cheap products are also the ones overconsumed in the United States and the ones that raise people's risk of developing obesity, heart disease, and type 2 diabetes. For more about the American food system, see Michael Pollan, *The Omnivore's Dilemma: A Natural History of Four Meals* (New York: Penguin, 2006), and Mark Bittman, *Animal, Vegetable, Junk: A History of Food, from Sustainable to Suicidal* (Boston: Houghton Mifflin Harcourt, 2021).

Big Food has also bought out plenty of scientists, nutritionists, dietitians, and universities. Research remains one of the food industry's most powerful marketing tactics. The industry funds scholars to conduct studies. When a medical journal publishes nutritional information resulting from studies that have been privately funded, the data appear objective; suddenly, marketing gets paraded as facts. This lack of transparency has been going on for decades—in 1967, the sugar industry paid three Harvard scientists the equivalent of about $50,000 in today's dollars to conduct research that proved sugar did not cause heart disease. The research, published in the prestigious *New England Journal of Medicine,* did not disclose industry funding. A 2013 analysis in the prestigious journal *PLOS Medicine* found that beverage studies funded by Coca-Cola, PepsiCo, the American Beverage Association, and the sugar industry were five times more likely *not* to find a link between sugary drinks and weight gain than studies whose authors reported no financial conflicts. Such conflicts of interest remain underreported, inconsistently described, and difficult to access.

For more information about how the food industry influences governmental nutritional recommendations and the nation's health, see Marion Nestle, *Food Politics: How the Food Industry Influences Nutrition and Health* (Berkeley: University of California Press, 2013). As she explains, "Many of the nutritional problems of Americans, not the least of them obesity, can be traced to the food industry's imperative to encourage people to eat more in order to generate sales and increase income." See also Jessica Almy and Margo Wootan, "Temptation at Checkout: The Food Industry's Sneaky Strategy for Selling More," Center for Science in the Public Interest (August 1, 2015).

6. As Tamar Haspel of the *Washington Post* argued, "Humans are simply ill-equipped to deal with a landscape of cheap, convenient, calorie-dense foods that have been specifically engineered to be irresistible. The inability to navigate our food environment is as near-universal as inabilities get"; see Tamar Haspel, "The True Connection Between Poverty and Obesity Isn't What You Probably Think," *Washington Post,* July 20, 2018.

7. For more information about differences in parent-child interactions around food across income levels, see Priya Fielding-Singh and Jennifer Wang, "Table Talk: How Mothers and Teenagers Across Socioeconomic Status Discuss Food," *Social Science and Medicine* 187 (August 2017): 49–57.

8. For more on Let's Move! and Michelle Obama's campaign to end childhood obesity, see Emily Wengrovius, "Healthy, Hunger-Free Kids Act of 2010 (P.L. 111-296) Summary," National Conference of State Legislatures, March 24, 2011, https://www.ncsl.org/research/human-services/healthy-hunger -free-kids-act-of-2010-summary.aspx; Hans Billger and Noereem Mena, "Make a Cafeteria Date to Eat a Healthy Lunch with Your Child at School," U.S. Department of Agriculture, February 21, 2017; Theresa Chalhoub et al., "Public Policies Promoting Healthy Eating and Exercise," Center for American Progress, November 27, 2018; "Healthy Food Financing Initiative," State of Childhood Obesity, Robert Wood Johnson Foundation, 2019.

9. Steven Cummins et al., "New Neighborhood Grocery Store Increased Awareness of Food Access but Did Not Alter Dietary Habits or Obesity," *Health Affairs* 33, no. 2 (February 2014): 283–91; Brian Elbel et al., "Assessment of a Government-Subsidized Supermarket in a High-Need

Area on Household Food Availability and Children's Dietary Intakes," *Public Health Nutrition* 18, no. 15 (October 2015): 2881–90. One interesting case occurred in Pittsburgh, where a study found that food-desert residents' diet quality and neighborhood satisfaction improved (although not their health outcomes) after a supermarket opened. Residents in the Pittsburgh study were actively involved in bringing a market to their neighborhood, with public discussions and marketing campaigns focusing on the need for healthy foods in the community. While the new supermarket may not have directly improved residents' diets, it likely had other positive impacts, as public and private investments stimulated economic development in the neighborhood and bolstered community members' morale. See Tamara Dubowitz et al., "Diet and Perceptions Change with Supermarket Introduction in a Food Desert, but Not Because of Supermarket Use," *Health Affairs* 34, no. 11 (2015): 1858–68, doi: 10.1377/hlthaff.2015.0667.

10. For more information on food access and food deserts, see Christine Byrne, "It's Great That We Talk About 'Food Deserts'—but It Might Be Time to Stop," *Huffington Post,* July 4, 2019; Michele Ver Ploeg et al., "Access to Affordable and Nutritious Food: Measuring and Understanding Food Deserts and Their Consequences: Report to Congress," U.S. Department of Agriculture, June 2009; Gina Kolata, "Studies Question the Pairing of Food Deserts and Obesity," *New York Times,* April 17, 2012. There are also differences of opinion about what constitutes food access. *New York Times* writer David Bornstein notes that "the standard way 'food deserts' have been defined may overemphasize—and in some cases mischaracterize—the problem of access and draw attention from other factors that influence what people buy and eat, like food prices, preparation time and knowledge, marketing, general levels of education, transportation, cultural practices and taste." Similarly, recent work over the past few years has emphasized the need to redefine what exactly is meant by *food access.* As public health scholars Donald Rose and Keelia O'Malley explain, the latest wave of food-access interventions has moved away from definitions based largely on purchasing power and geographic location and moved toward ones that see "the problem as structural in nature, originating in socially determined inequities." Organizations intervening under these new definitions "use the food system as an entry point, but they cut across various sectors—education, employment, community development, business development, agriculture, environment, and health." See David Bornstein, "Time to Revisit Food Deserts," *New York Times,* April 25, 2012; Donald Rose and Keelia O'Malley, "Food Access 3.0: Insights from Post-Katrina New Orleans on an Evolving Approach to Food Inequities," *American Journal of Public Health* 110 (2020): 1495–97.

11. This does not mean that geographic food access is never an issue. My conclusion relates to a suburban setting in one area of the country with a nonrandom sample of families. Rural regions, urban areas, American

Indian reservations—these are places where food access may be more challenging and exert a greater influence on people's diets.

12. That said, average distances are slightly shorter among low-income households (4.8 miles) and slightly longer among households living in food deserts (nearly 7 miles). Still, the takeaway holds. See Hunt Allcott et al., "Food Deserts and the Causes of Nutritional Inequality," *Quarterly Journal of Economics* 134, no. 4 (November 2019): 1793–1844, https://doi -org.stanford.idm.oclc.org/10.1093/qje/qjz015.

13. "Poorest US Households Spent 33% of Their Incomes on Food in 2015," *FreshPlaza*, May 24, 2017, www.freshplaza.com/article/2175991/poorest -us-households-spent-33-of-their-incomes-on-food-in-2015/.

14. For more information on SNAP, see "Policy Basics: The Supplemental Nutrition Assistance Program (SNAP)," Center on Budget and Policy Priorities, June 25, 2019, www.cbpp.org/research/food-assistance/policy -basics-the-supplemental-nutrition-assistance-program-snap.

15. Steven Carlson, "More Adequate SNAP Benefits Would Help Millions of Participants Better Afford Food," Center on Budget and Policy Priorities, July 30, 2019.

16. Marge Dwyer, "Eating Healthy vs. Unhealthy Diet Costs About $1.50 More per Day," Harvard T. H. Chan School of Public Health, January 13, 2014, https://www.hsph.harvard.edu/news/press-releases/healthy-vs -unhealthy-diet-costs-1-50-more/.

17. How much families spent on food varied each month. The typical source of variation was whether and how much families ate out. Grocery-store expenses were more consistent. These estimates are based on the months I observed each family.

18. In California, SNAP is known as CalFresh. CalFresh income eligibility rates are determined by family size, income, and some living costs. Individuals can have income from a full- or part-time job, unemployment benefits, General Relief, or CalWORKs (a public assistance program that provides cash aid and services to eligible families that have children in the home) and still get CalFresh. In 2019–2020, a household of one was eligible for CalFresh if its gross monthly income did not exceed $1,354, and the maximum SNAP benefit amount was $194. A household of two could not have a monthly income over $1,832, and the maximum benefit was $355. A household of three could not earn over $2,311, and the maximum benefit was $509. Households may have up to $2,250 in countable resources (such as cash or money in a bank account) and still be eligible. SNAP eligibility has never been extended to undocumented noncitizens. The Food and Nutrition Act of 2008 limits eligibility for SNAP benefits to U.S. citizens and certain lawfully present noncitizens. Generally, to qualify for SNAP, noncitizens must have lived in the United States for at least five years, receive disability-related assistance or benefits, or be a child under eighteen.

19. Public programs like food stamps incentivize living alone. Larger households receive more in food stamps but not as much as members of

that household would receive if they lived separately. When Marcus applied on his own, he got the maximum benefit amount of $194. What was confusing about Nyah's situation was that she didn't then separately apply for SNAP. If she had, she would have also qualified for between $150 and $194, bringing their grand total to just under $400. I believe she held off on applying for SNAP because she was waiting to get SSI, which would then have covered some of her food costs. Nyah once told me, "I have no income, but they're trying to put me on SSI."

20. Until June 2019, California residents who received SSI were not eligible to receive SNAP because California gave these SSI recipients extra money to be used for food. This was the case for Mariah and Natasha; they did not qualify for SNAP funds, as their SSI allotments were intended to pay for some food. It was never clear to me if Nyah knew this. She once told me, "My kids, they don't care about food stamps because they get SSI and they don't need that." Regardless, Nyah did put some of the money they received toward food.

21. "The Impact of the Coronavirus on Food Insecurity in 2020 and 2021," Feeding America, March 31, 2021, https://www.feedingamerica.org /research/coronavirus-hunger-research.

22. D. W. Schanzenbach and A. Pitts, "How Much Has Food Insecurity Risen? Evidence from the Census Household Pulse Survey," Institute for Policy Research, Northwestern University, June 10, 2020, https://www .ipr.northwestern.edu/documents/reports/ipr-rapid-researchreports -pulse-hh-data-10-june-2020.pdf.

23. Cindy W. Leung et al., "Food Insecurity Is Inversely Associated with Diet Quality of Lower-Income Adults," *Journal of the Academy of Nutrition and Dietetics* 114, no. 12 (December 2014): 1943–53.

24. Emma J. Stinson et al., "Food Insecurity Is Associated with Maladaptive Eating Behaviors and Objectively Measured Overeating," *Obesity* 26, no. 12 (2018): 1841–48.

Chapter 4: All That Matters

1. While mothers' accounts diverged from prevailing public health narratives, these accounts were consistent with findings from sociological studies of families living in poverty. Two stand out. First, Kathryn Edin and Laura Lein found in their research on single, low-income mothers that these mothers occasionally forgo material necessities in order to pay for a trip to fast-food restaurants or other types of culinary treats for their children. Second, in his ethnographic study of eviction, Matthew Desmond tells the story of a low-income woman who spends all of her food stamps for a month on one meal of lobster tails, shrimp, king crab legs, salad, and lemon meringue pie. See Kathryn Edin and Laura Lein, *Making Ends Meet: How Single Mothers Survive Welfare and Low-Wage Work* (New York: Russell Sage Foundation, 1997); Matthew Desmond, *Evicted: Profit and Poverty in the American City* (New York: Crown, 2016).

2. For more about food's symbolic value to low-income mothers, see Priya Fielding-Singh, "A Taste of Inequality: Food's Symbolic Value Across the Socioeconomic Spectrum," *Sociological Science* (August 2017).

Chapter 5: Scarcity, Abundance

1. For more information about migration and segregation patterns in the Bay Area, see Stephen Menendian and Samir Gambhir, "Racial Segregation in the San Francisco Bay Area," Othering and Belonging Institute, 2018, https://belonging.berkeley.edu/segregationinthebay, and Tony Roshan Samara, "Race, Inequality, and the Resegregation of the Bay Area," Urban Habitat, 2016, http://urbanhabitat.org/sites/default/files/UH%20Policy%20Brief2016.pdf.

Chapter 6: Within Reach

1. For more information about the culture-of-poverty argument, see Phillippe Bourgois, "Culture of Poverty," in *International Encyclopedia of the Social and Behavioral Sciences*, 2nd ed., ed. James Wright (Amsterdam: Elsevier, 2015); Judith Goode and Edwin Eames, "An Anthropological Critique of the Culture of Poverty," in *Urban Life*, ed. G. Gmelch and W. Zenner (Long Grove, IL: Waveland, 1996). For a more relevant and attuned discussion of the relationship between culture and poverty, see Mario Luis Small, David J. Harding, and Michèle Lamont, "Reconsidering Culture and Poverty," *Annals of the American Academy of Political and Social Science* 629, no. 1 (2010): 6–27.

2. For a discussion of the 2020 Lawrence Mead paper, see Colleen Flaherty, "U.S. and Them," *Inside Higher Ed*, July 28, 2020; "News Release: Statement from Faculty of Arts and Science and Wagner Leadership Regarding Professor Lawrence Mead," New York University, July 27, 2020, https://www.nyu.edu/about/news-publications/news/2020/july/Statement_FAS_Wagner_Leadership_Lawrence_Mead.html.

3. Allison J. Pugh, "Windfall Child Rearing: Low-Income Care and Consumption," *Journal of Consumer Culture* 4, no. 2 (2004): 229–49. As Matthew Desmond writes, "To Sammy, Pastor Dayle and others, Larraine was poor because she threw money away. But the reverse was more true. Larraine threw money away because she was poor"; see Matthew Desmond, *Evicted: Profit and Poverty in the American City* (New York: Crown, 2016), 219.

4. This insight also aligns with that of Allison Pugh in *Longing and Belonging: Parents, Children and Consumer Culture*, in which she draws on her ethnographic study of how parents from different socioeconomic backgrounds navigate consumer culture. Pugh demonstrates how families from different class backgrounds differentially engage in and rationalize consumption choices for their children. While affluent families engage in a process of "symbolic deprivation," Pugh finds that low-income families engage in "symbolic indulgence." The affluent families in Pugh's study pointed to goods or experiences that their children did not have as evidence

of their own moral restraint and worthiness as parents. In contrast, low-income parents sometimes made considerable sacrifices to ensure that their children had particular goods or experiences, often prioritizing their children's needs over their own. In these families, it was important to the parents to demonstrate that their children were not missing out because of their socioeconomic position; it was important for parents that their kids felt "normal." See A. J. Pugh, *Longing and Belonging: Parents, Children and Consumer Culture* (Berkeley: University of California Press, 2009).

Chapter 7: Being "Good"

1. "Survey: Moms Still Make Most Household Purchase Decisions," *Chain Store Age,* October 24, 2013; "What Busy Moms Sneak In... TV Time," *Wall Street Journal,* November 2011.

2. Moms today are up against food and beverage industries that target children, a vulnerable, susceptible, and profitable audience for marketing. Although many countries around the world tightly control or ban food advertising and marketing aimed at youth, the United States has not done that since 1980, when, in response to corporate pressure, Congress removed the Federal Trade Commission's authority to restrict food advertising and limited its jurisdiction regarding advertising to children. Marketing campaigns targeting kids are extremely effective at making them want to eat more high-calorie, unhealthy products. The marketing is also masterfully placed. There's a reason why the least healthy products in supermarkets—those often plastered with words in kid-friendly fonts and cartoon characters—are located right at or just below children's eye level. The industry adage that "eye level is buy level" captures this strategy of marketing directly to the kids themselves. Madison and Paige used their "pester power" to wear Dana down to get the stuff they craved.

   In 2016, the television ads aimed at children primarily promoted unhealthy products, including fast food, candy, sweet and salty snacks, and sugary drinks; fewer than 10 percent of food ads promoted healthier products. Young kids' developing brains prevent them from discerning advertising from truth, which has led both the American Psychological Association and American Academy of Pediatrics to call marketing to children under eight inherently unfair and deceptive. But even teens and young adults are tricked by food and beverage marketing; product placements are skillfully and subtly woven into video games, movies, and social media posts by celebrities and influencers on Instagram, Twitter, and YouTube.

   For more about the food industry's marketing tactics and impacts, see Michael Moss, *Salt Sugar Fat: How the Food Giants Hooked Us* (New York: Random House, 2013); Michael Moss, *Hooked: Free Will, and How the Food Giants Exploit Our Addictions* (New York: Random House, 2021); B. Sadeghirad et al., "Influence of Unhealthy Food and Beverage

Marketing on Children's Dietary Intake and Preference: A Systematic Review and Meta-Analysis of Randomized Trials," *Obesity Reviews* 17, no. 10 (October 2016): 945–59.

For more about the food industry's marketing specifically to children, see Jennifer Harris et al., "Food Industry Self-Regulation After 10 Years: Progress and Opportunities to Improve Food Advertising to Children," Rudd Center for Food Policy and Obesity (2017); Bettina Siegel, *Kid Food: The Challenge of Feeding Children in a Highly Processed World* (New York: Oxford University Press, 2019); J. A. Horsley et al., "The Proportion of Unhealthy Foodstuffs Children Are Exposed to at the Checkout of Convenience Supermarkets," *Public Health Nutrition* 17, no. 11 (November 2014): 2453–58.

3. For more about intensive mothering, see Sharon Hays, *The Cultural Contradictions of Motherhood* (New Haven, CT: Yale University Press, 1996); Deirdre Johnston and Debra Swanson, "Constructing the 'Good Mother': The Experience of Mothering Ideologies by Work Status," *Sex Roles* 54 (2006): 509–19; Paula K. McDonald, Lisa M. Bradley, and Diane Guthrie, "Good Mothers, Bad Mothers: Exploring the Relationship Between Attitudes Towards Nonmaternal Childcare and Mothers' Labour Force Participation," *Journal of Family Studies* 11 (2005): 62–82; J. A. Reich, "Neoliberal Mothering and Vaccine Refusal: Imagined Gated Communities and the Privilege of Choice," *Gender and Society* 28, no. 5 (2014): 679–704.

Recent work highlights that mothers of color and employed, low-income, and single mothers experience and interpret motherhood differently than white, class-privileged, married mothers. This research has generated offshoots of the intensive-mothering ideology that highlight such critical differences; these include extensive mothering, integrated mothering, defensive mothering, and inventive mothering. Key differences between these ideologies and that of intensive mothering pertain to mothers' varying attitudes toward and practices related to family, child-rearing, and motherhood. See Karen Christopher, "Extensive Mothering: Employed Mothers' Constructions of the Good Mother," *Gender and Society* 26, no. 1 (2012): 73–96; D. M. Dow, "Integrated Motherhood: Beyond Hegemonic Ideologies of Motherhood," *Journal of Marriage and Family* 78 (February 2016): 180–96; S. Elliott and S. Bowen, "Defending Motherhood: Morality, Responsibility, and Double Binds in Feeding Children," *Journal of Marriage and Family* 80 (April 2018): 499–520; Patricia Hill Collins, *Black Feminist Thought: Knowledge, Consciousness, and the Politics of Empowerment* (Boston: Unwin Hyman, 1990); Jennifer Randles, "Willing to Do Anything for My Kids: Inventive Mothering, Diapers, and the Inequalities of Carework," *American Sociological Review* 86, no. 1 (2021): 35–59.

Christopher's 2012 study of working mothers reveals that under an extensive-mothering ideal, mothers redefine *good mothering* as being "in charge" and responsible for children's well-being even when mothers are not providing that care as well as limiting the infringement of employment on family life. In her study of Black middle-class mothers, Dow finds that their adherence to an integrated-mothering ideology means that they see child-rearing, while mother-centered, as extended-family- and community-supported. This collective responsibility for children aligns with Collins's argument that Black communities have "recognized that vesting one person with full responsibility for mothering a child may not be wise or possible." As a result, other women—grandmothers and other extended family who assist by sharing mothering responsibilities—traditionally have been central to the institution of Black motherhood. Dow also finds that mothers view working outside the home as a duty of motherhood rather than a selfish sacrifice. Elliott and Bowen leverage intensive mothering and the conceptualization of defensive othering to define defensive mothering as the strategy that low-income mothers of color engage in to present themselves as responsible, caring, informed mothers and deflect negative characterizations of their mothering in the face of societal scrutiny and surveillance. All of this research on diverse experiences and ideological variations of motherhood highlights that, as widespread as intensive-mothering norms may be in the U.S., there exists no uniform interpretation or performance of the ideal.

At the same time, these studies highlight that whatever variations exist, two transcending tenets underpin what it means to be a good mother in the U.S. First, all ideals—intensive, extensive, integrated, and defensive— maintain that child-rearing is a generally mother-centered activity that demands devoting resources—often time, energy, and money—to children. Second, while not all mothers navigate or perform the same mothering practices, intensive mothering is still the normative standard by which mothering is societally assessed in Western contexts. That is, whatever ideals mothers internally subscribe to or externally perform, they are nonetheless societally judged by the standard of intensive mothering.

4. Caitlin Collins, *Making Motherhood Work: How Women Manage Careers and Caregiving* (Princeton, NJ: Princeton University Press, 2019).

5. Patrick Ishizuka, "Social Class, Gender, and Contemporary Parenting Standards in the United States: Evidence from a National Survey Experiment," *Social Forces* 98, no. 1 (September 2019): 31–58; Jennifer Lois, "The Temporal Emotion Work of Motherhood: Homeschoolers' Strategies for Managing Time Shortage," *Gender and Society* 24, no. 4 (2010): 421–46.

6. For more on the centrality of food to motherhood, see Joslyn Brenton, "The Limits of Intensive Feeding: Maternal Foodwork at the Intersection of Race, Class, and Gender," *Sociology of Health and Illness* 39, no. 6 (2017): 863–77; Kate Cairns, Josée Johnston, and Merin Oleschuk, "Calibrating Motherhood," in *Feeding Children Inside and Outside the Home: Critical Perspectives,* ed. V. Harman, B. Cappellini, and C. Faircloth (New York: Routledge, 2019); Merin Oleschuk, "Gender, Cultural Schemas and Learning to Cook," *Gender and Society* 33 no. 4 (2019): 607–28; Kate

Cairns and Josée Johnston, *Food and Femininities* (London: Bloomsbury, 2015).

Chapter 8: Hunger and Pickiness

1. Also see Caitlin Daniel, "Economic Constraints on Taste Formation and the True Cost of Healthy Eating," *Social Science and Medicine* 148 (2016): 34–41.

2. For more about Smart Snacks, see Jennifer L. Harris et al., "Effects of Offering Look-Alike Products as Smart Snacks in Schools," *Childhood Obesity* 12, no. 6 (2016): 432–39.

3. Delfina made around $2,400 a month as a cashier, but she also received $500 a month in child support and, eventually, another $1,000 in rental income from the house her parents purchased back in 1980. That brought her monthly income to around $3,900 and her yearly income to $48,000. When Luis was in elementary school, Delfina learned that her total income made him ineligible for free or reduced school lunch. She could not believe it, but after that discovery she never again checked to see if he was eligible. SNAP eligibility guidelines suggest that he would not have been eligible, as the monthly income cap for a household of two is $1,832. Because lunch was not free at school, Delfina sent Luis with the few dollars it cost each day to purchase the cafeteria lunch, which he generally did not buy.

4. Michelle Chen, "Nearly 1 in 3 Restaurant Workers Suffers from Food Insecurity," *Nation,* July 30, 2014.

5. For more information about the organic child ideal and the pressures of ethical consumption, see Kate Cairns, Josée Johnston, and Norah MacKendrick, "Feeding the 'Organic Child': Mothering Through Ethical Consumption," *Journal of Consumer Culture* 13, no. 2 (2013): 97–118; Kate Cairns, Norah MacKendrick, and Josée Johnston, "The 'Organic Child' Ideal Holds Mothers to an Impossible Standard," *Aeon*, February 19, 2020; Kate Cairns and Josée Johnston, "On (Not) Knowing Where Your Food Comes From: Meat, Mothering and Ethical Eating," *Agriculture and Human Values* 35 (2018): 569–80; Josée Johnston and Shyon Baumann, *Foodies: Democracy and Distinction in the Gourmet Foodscape* (New York: Routledge, 2010); Norah MacKendrick, "More Work for Mother: Chemical Body Burdens as a Maternal Responsibility," *Gender and Society* 28 (2014): 705–28.

Chapter 10: Kale Salad

1. It's telling that Southern cuisine and soul food are believed to be a major cause of higher rates of type 2 diabetes and hypertension within Black communities even though research points more convincingly to other causes, such as environmental racism, discrimination, stress, and poor health-care access and quality. See Maanvi Singh, "Southern Diet Blamed for High Rates of Hypertension Among Black Americans," *The Salt* (blog), NPR, October 2, 2018; Psyche Williams-Forson, "More Than

Just the 'Big Piece of Chicken': The Power of Race, Class, and Food in American Consciousness," in *Food and Culture: A Reader,* 2nd ed., ed. C. Counihan and P. van Esterik (New York: Routledge, 2007), 107–17.

2. For more about diet culture and racism in America, see Sabrina Strings, *Fearing the Black Body: The Racial Origins of Fat Phobia* (New York: New York University Press, 2019); Priya Krishna, "Is American Dietetics a White-Bread World? These Dieticians Think So," *New York Times,* December 7, 2020; Nicole Danielle Schott, "Race, Online Space and the Feminine: Unmapping 'Black Girl Thinspiration,'" *Critical Sociology* 43, nos. 7–8 (2017): 1029–43; Hanna Garth and Ashanté M. Reese, eds., *Black Food Matters: Racial Justice in the Wake of Food Justice* (Minneapolis: University of Minnesota Press, 2020).

3. Rebekah Kebede, "Collards vs. Kale: Why Only One Supergreen Is a Superstar," *National Geographic,* October 12, 2016.

Chapter 11: Mom's Job

1. Katherine Schaeffer, "Among U.S. Couples, Women Do More Cooking and Grocery Shopping than Men," Pew Research Center, September 24, 2019.

2. D'Vera Cohn and Jeffrey S. Passel, "A Record 64 Million Americans Live in Multigenerational Households," Pew Research Center, April 5, 2018, https://www.pewresearch.org/fact-tank/2018/04/05/a-record-64-million-americans-live-in-multigenerational-households/.

3. Schaeffer, "Among U.S. Couples."

4. While I don't go into depth about these outliers in this book, other research examines the experiences and perspectives of men with significant domestic cooking responsibilities. This research finds that such men may frame meal planning and cooking in traditionally feminine terms. For instance, using interviews, cooking observations, and meal diaries from thirty such men in Canada, the sociologist Michelle Szabo found that these men view cooking as a form of care and concern for the family's satisfaction and health. See Michelle Szabo, "Men Nurturing Through Food: Challenging Gender Dichotomies Around Domestic Cooking," *Journal of Gender Studies* 23, no. 1 (2014): 18–31.

This work also underscores how constructions of masculinity and fatherhood are not fixed but can be negotiated and challenged. Broader sociopolitical structures and social norms can help incorporate domestic investments in foodwork into men's sense of masculinity. For instance, research conducted in Sweden, a national context where domestic labor has become increasingly de-gendered, shows that with gender-equal policies and public discourses, foodwork can become not only legitimate and expected for men but also incorporated into men's expressions of progressive masculinity. See Nicklas Neuman, Lucas Gottzén, and Christina Fjellström, "Narratives of Progress: Cooking and Gender Equality Among Swedish Men," *Journal of Gender Studies* (2015): 1–13.

5. Research in the United States and United Kingdom on mothers' views on fathers' involvement in foodwork shows that mothers characterize fathers as uninvolved or tangential to this work. When fathers do contribute to feeding families, they do so in a mostly supportive role, acting as sous-chefs and helping with special occasion cooking. See J. Blissett, C. Meyer, and E. Haycraft, "Maternal and Paternal Controlling Feeding Practices with Male and Female Children," *Appetite* 47, no. 2 (2006): 212–19; Kate Cairns, Josée Johnston, and Norah MacKendrick, "Feeding the 'Organic Child': Mothering Through Ethical Consumption," *Journal of Consumer Culture* 13, no. 2 (2013): 97–118; Rebecca O'Connell and Julia Brannen, *Food, Families and Work* (London: Bloomsbury, 2016); Brenda Beagan et al., " 'It's Just Easier for Me to Do It': Rationalizing the Family Division of Foodwork," *Sociology* 42, no. 4 (2008): 653–71.

6. While many moms (and dads) may feel that moms have a unique expertise when it comes to kids' diets, Sharon Hays, in *The Cultural Contradictions of Motherhood* (New Haven, CT: Yale University Press, 1996), 72, reminds us that it is "difficult to distinguish a 'mother's intuition' from ideas arising from a woman's social role, a woman's upbringing, and the culture of motherhood."

7. For more about the expectations of modern fatherhood and the centrality of food to motherhood and femininity as well as its peripherality to fatherhood, see Marjorie DeVault, *Feeding the Family: The Social Organization of Caring as Gendered Work* (Chicago: University of Chicago Press, 1994); Caron Bove and Jeffery Sobal, "Foodwork in Newly Married Couples: Making Family Meals," *Food, Culture and Society* 9, no. 1 (2006): 70–89; Caron Bove, Jeffery Sobal, and Barbara Rauschenbach, "Food Choices Among Newly Married Couples: Convergence, Conflict, Individualism, and Projects," *Appetite* 40, no. 1 (2003): 25–41.

8. For more about how conventional masculinity norms can discourage fathers from engaging in healthy behaviors, including healthy eating, see Will H. Courtenay, "Constructions of Masculinity and Their Influence on Men's Well-Being: A Theory of Gender and Health," *Social Science and Medicine* 50, no. 10 (2000): 1385–1401; David Williams, "The Health of Men: Structured Inequalities and Opportunities," *American Journal of Public Health* 93 (2003): 724–31. For more about masculinity and dietary consumption, see Carrie R. Daniel et al., "Trends in Meat Consumption in the United States," *Public Health and Nutrition* 14, no. 4 (2011): 575–83; Matthew B. Ruby and Steven J. Heine, "Meat, Morals and Masculinity," *Appetite* 56, no. 2 (2011): 447–50; Sandra Nakagawa and Chloe Grace Hart, "Where's the Beef? How Masculinity Exacerbates Gender Disparities in Health Behaviors," *Socius* (2019).

9. I write more elsewhere about the role of fathers in family food practices, as well as how fathers' dietary approaches reflect and reinforce traditional gender norms and expectations within families. See Priya Fielding-Singh, "Dining with Dad: Fathers' Influences on Family Food Practices," *Appetite* 117 (October 2017): 98–108.

10. In the United States, the unequal distribution of food labor holds, regardless of maternal employment status; that is, even within families where both parents are employed full-time, mothers continue to shoulder most of the foodwork responsibilities. See Jill E. Yavorsky, Claire M. Kamp Dush, and Sarah J. Schoppe-Sullivan, "The Production of Inequality: The Gender Division of Labor Across the Transition to Parenthood," *Family Relations* 77 (2015): 662–79; Jennifer Hook, "Gender Inequality in the Welfare State: Sex Segregation in Housework, 1965–2003," *American Journal of Sociology* 115, no. 5 (2010): 1480–1523.

Chapter 12: Time and Money

1. In their 2019 book, the sociologists Sarah Bowen, Joslyn Brenton, and Sinikka Elliott show the pressures mothers are under to provide home-cooked meals and the challenges they face in doing so, highlighting how modern families struggle to confront high expectations and deep-seated inequalities around getting food on the table. They critique widespread messages advocated by foodies and public health officials that reforming the food system requires a return to the kitchen. They argue that time pressures, money-saving trade-offs, and gendered norms of pleasing others make it nearly impossible for mothers to achieve the idealized vision of home-cooked meals. See Sarah Bowen, Joslyn Brenton, and Sinikka Elliott, *Pressure Cooker: Why Home Cooking Won't Solve Our Problems and What We Can Do About It* (New York: Oxford University Press, 2019); Sarah Bowen, Sinikka Elliott, and Joslyn Brenton, "The Joy of Cooking?," *Contexts* 13, no. 3 (2014): 20–25.

   Relatedly, the sociologist Merin Oleschuk finds, in her analysis of North American news media representations of family meals, that while the media largely trace the "demise" of the family meal to structural causes, they focus on individual solutions and overemphasize the agency and responsibility of individuals—namely, mothers—for restoring the family meal. As Oleschuk explains, "Despite determining that the reasons families are not cooking enough is complex, news media conclude that parents (largely mothers) must simply work harder to do so." See Merin Oleschuk, "In Today's Market, Your Food Chooses You: News Media Constructions of Responsibility for Health Through Cooking," *Social Problems* 67, no. 1 (2020): 3.

2. Gretchen Livingston, "It's No Longer a 'Leave It to Beaver' World for American Families—but It Wasn't Back Then, Either," Pew Research Center, December 30, 2015, https://www.pewresearch.org/fact-tank /2015/12/30/its-no-longer-a-leave-it-to-beaver-world-for-american -families-but-it-wasnt-back-then-either/.

3. Lisa Valente, "How to Eat Healthy When You Don't Have Time to Meal Prep," *Eating Well*, September 6, 2018; John Rampton, "Twelve Ways to Eat Healthy No Matter How Busy You Are," *Entrepreneur*, May 5, 2015; Ellie Krieger, *Weeknight Wonders: Delicious, Healthy Dinners in Thirty Minutes or Less* (Boston: Houghton Mifflin Harcourt, 2013); Carrie

Forrest, *The Quick and Easy Healthy Cookbook* (Emeryville, CA: Rockridge Press, 2019); Carrie Madormo, "Seventy-Two Easy Kid-Friendly Dinners Perfect for Weeknights," *Taste of Home* (blog), July 30, 2020; Amy Palanjian, "A Week of Healthy Kids Meal Ideas (That Actually Work in Real Life)," *Yummy Toddler Food* (blog), August 18, 2020.

4. When I spoke with Arjun and Sonali later, I learned that this solution had turned out to be a long-term one. They continued to employ their cook for years after I met them (although they stopped in March 2020 in light of the COVID-19 shelter-in-place orders).

Chapter 14: Fluctuating Finances

1. See Anne Helen Petersen, "America's Hollow Middle Class," *Vox*, December 15, 2020; "America's Shrinking Middle Class: A Close Look at Changes Within Metropolitan Areas," Pew Research Center, May 11, 2016.

Chapter 15: Becoming American

1. Increased acculturation to the United States is associated with decreased dietary quality, in particular increased consumption of dietary fat and decreased consumption of fruits and vegetables. See J. Satia-Abouta et al., "Dietary Acculturation: Applications to Nutrition Research and Dietetics," *Journal of the American Dietetic Association* 102 (2002): 1105–18, and I. A. Lesser, D. Gasevic, and S. A. Lear, "The Association Between Acculturation and Dietary Patterns of South Asian Immigrants," *PLOS One* 9, no. 2 (2014): e88495.

This is particularly true among Latinx immigrants, whose kids' diets decrease in quality over time in the U.S. See J. Van Hook et al., "It Is Hard to Swim Upstream: Dietary Acculturation Among Mexican-Origin Children," *Population Research and Policy Review* 35, no. 2 (2016): 177–96; Ji-Hong Liu et al., "Generation and Acculturation Status Are Associated with Dietary Intake and Body Weight in Mexican American Adolescents," *Journal of Nutrition* 142, no. 2 (2012): 298–305.

Chapter 16: Downscaling

1. See K. Leifheit et al., "Eviction in the United States: Affected Populations, Housing and Neighborhood-Level Consequences, and Implications for Health," Society for Epidemiologic Research Meeting, 2018; M. Desmond and R. Kimbro, "Eviction's Fallout: Housing, Hardship, and Health," *Social Forces* 94, no. 1 (2015): 295–324, doi:10.1093/sf/sov044.

2. Arlie Russell Hochschild, "Emotion Work, Feeling Rules, and Social Structure," *American Journal of Sociology* 85 (1979): 551–75.

3. Marianne Cooper, *Cut Adrift: Families in Insecure Times* (Berkeley: University of California Press, 2014).

4. For more about the mediating role of stress in the connection between poverty and health, see L. I. Pearlin, "The Sociological Study of Stress," *Journal of Health and Social Behavior* 30 (1989): 241–56; D. M.

Almeida et al., "Do Daily Stress Processes Account for Socioeconomic Health Disparities?," *Journal of Gerontology* 60 (2005): 34–39; J. Kahn and L. I. Pearlin, "Financial Strain Over the Life Course and Health Among Older Adults," *Journal of Health and Social Behavior* 47 (2006): 17–31; B. S. McEwen, "Protective and Damaging Effects of Stress Mediators," *New England Journal of Medicine* 338 (1998): 171–79.

Chapter 17: Upscaling

1. For more about the anxiety that characterizes modern parenting, see Claire Cain Miller, "The Relentlessness of Modern Parenting," *New York Times*, December 25, 2018; Jessica Calarco, *Negotiating Opportunities: How the Middle Class Secures Advantages in School* (New York: Oxford University Press, 2018); Suzanne M. Bianchi, John P. Robinson, and Melissa A. Milkie, *Changing Rhythms of American Family Life* (New York: Russell Sage Foundation, 2006); Susan Shaw, "Family Leisure and Changing Ideologies of Parenthood," *Sociology Compass* 2, no. 2 (2008): 688–703.

2. Gretchen Livingston, "Stay-at-Home Moms and Dads Account for About One-in-Five U.S. Parents," Pew Research Center, September 24, 2018.

Chapter 18: Priorities

1. This echoes national research, which shows that intimate-partner violence rates are highest in the poorest neighborhoods. Similarly, residential segregation causes low-income families to live in neighborhoods where disadvantage is concentrated, with poorer-quality schools, more environmental hazards, and less safe outdoor spaces. See C. R. Browning, "The Span of Collective Efficacy: Extending Social Disorganization Theory to Partner Violence," *Journal of Marriage and Family* 64 (2002): 833–50; G. L. Fox and M. L. Benson, "Household and Neighborhood Contexts of Intimate Partner Violence," *Public Health Reports* 121 (2006): 419–27; P. O'Campo et al., "Violence by Male Partners Against Women During the Childbearing Year: A Contextual Analysis," *American Journal of Public Health* 85 (1995): 1092–97; Vanessa Sacks, "Five Ways Neighborhoods of Concentrated Disadvantage Harm Children," Child Trends, February 14, 2018, www.childtrends.org/child-trends-5/five-ways-neighborhoods-concentrated-disadvantage-harm-children.

Chapter 19: Control

1. For more about the rug rat race, see Garey Ramey and Valerie A. Ramey, "The Rug Rat Race," *Brookings Papers on Economic Activity* 41 (Spring 2010): 129–99, and W. Bentley MacLeod and Miguel Urquiola, "Reputation and School Competition," *American Economic Review* 105 (2015): 3471–88.

2. For more about these forms of parenting, see Claire Cain Miller and Jonah Engel Bromwich, "How Parents Are Robbing Their Children of Adulthood," *New York Times*, March 16, 2019; Ben Zimmer,

" 'Snowplowing': When Parents Try to Clear All Obstacles," *Wall Street Journal,* March 29, 2019; Erin Leonard, "Snow Plowing Plows a Child's Character," *Psychology Today,* March 26, 2019.

It's also worth noting that as well intentioned as these parents' efforts may be, they have downsides, most notably kids' mental health. More advantaged teenagers report higher rates of alcohol and drug abuse than lower-income teens and clinically significant depression or anxiety at two to three times the rate of the national average. For more information, see S. S. Luthar, P. J. Small, and L. Ciciolla, "Adolescents from Upper Middle Class Communities: Substance Misuse and Addiction Across Early Adulthood," *Development and Psychopathology* 30, no. 1 (2018): 315–35. In the Bay Area, a place of tremendously high academic standards and tough competition for admission into top colleges and universities, there was a string of student suicides at top high schools in the area during the time of this research. These suicides inspired local and national conversation about the stresses and pressures parents were inflicting on their kids in the hopes of ensuring their success to the detriment of students' mental health and well-being. For more information, see Hanna Rosin, "The Silicon Valley Suicides," *Atlantic,* December 2015.

3. For more about concerted cultivation and the accomplishment of natural growth, see Annette Lareau, *Unequal Childhoods* (Berkeley: University of California Press, 2003).

Chapter 21: Windfall

1. For more about paying families for participating in observations, see Annette Lareau and Aliya Hamid Rao, "Intensive Family Observations: A Methodological Guide," *Sociological Methods and Research* (April 2020).

Chapter 22: Where We Go

1. My foster siblings' names have been replaced with pseudonyms, and their identifying characteristics have been changed.
2. See Priya Fielding-Singh, "Dining with Dad: Fathers' Influences on Family Food Practices," *Appetite* 117 (October 2017): 98–108, and Priya Fielding-Singh, "Fathers Should Take More Active Role in Families' Healthy Eating," *San Francisco Chronicle,* July 17, 2017.
3. Colin Gray, "Leaving Benefits on the Table: Evidence from SNAP," *Journal of Public Economics* 179 (November 2019): 104054.
4. Patricia M. Anderson et al., "Beyond Income: What Else Predicts Very Low Food Security Among Children?," *Southern Economic Journal* 82, no. 4 (2016): 1078–1105, doi: 10.1002/soej.12079.
5. Fang Zhang et al., "Trends and Disparities in Diet Quality Among US Adults by Supplemental Nutrition Assistance Program Participation Status," *JAMA Network Open* 1, no. 2 (2018).
6. Patricia Anderson and Kristin Butcher, "The Relationships Among SNAP Benefits, Grocery Spending, Diet Quality, and the Adequacy of

Low-Income Families' Resources," Center on Budget and Policy Priorities, June 14, 2016, www.cbpp.org/research/food-assistance/the-relationships -among-snap-benefits-grocery-spending-diet-quality-and-the.

7. "Supplemental Nutrition Assistance Program: Initiatives to Make SNAP Benefits More Adequate Significantly Improve Food Security, Nutrition, and Health," Food Research and Action Center, February 2019, https:// frac.org/research/resource-library/supplemental-nutrition-assistance -program-initiatives-to-make-snap-benefits-more-adequate-significantly -improve-food-security-nutrition-and-health; Carrie M. Durward et al., "Double Up Food Bucks Participation Is Associated with Increased Fruit and Vegetable Consumption and Food Security Among Low-Income Adults," *Journal of Nutrition Education and Behavior* 51, no. 3 (October 16, 2018): 342–47; "Food Insecurity Nutrition Incentive Program (FINI)," 2015 program results, Farmers Market Coalition, 2017.

8. "School Nutrition," Centers for Disease Control and Prevention, page last reviewed February 15, 2021.

9. Amy Ellen Schwartz and Micah W. Rothbart, "Let Them Eat Lunch: The Impact of Universal Free Meals on Student Performance," *Center for Policy Research* 235 (Fall 2017).

10. Jennifer L. Harris and Tracy Fox, "Food and Beverage Marketing in Schools: Putting Student Health at the Head of the Class," *JAMA Pediatrics* 168, no. 3 (2014): 206–208.

11. A 2015 survey by the Rudd Center for Food Policy and Obesity surveyed over 3,600 parents and found that approximately 4 in 5 agreed that food companies should reduce marketing unhealthy foods and drinks to kids and 2 in 3 believed that food companies make it difficult for parents to raise healthy kids. See Jennifer Harris et al., "Parents' Attitudes About Food Marketing to Children: 2012 to 2015 Opportunities and Challenges to Creating Demand for a Healthier Food Environment," Rudd Center for Food Policy and Obesity, April 2017.

12. For more about the unaffordability of housing in America, see Matthew Desmond, "Unaffordable America: Poverty, Housing, and Eviction," *Fast Focus: Institute for Research on Poverty* 22 (March 2015): 1–6; Laurie Goodman and Bhargavi Ganesh, "Low-Income Homeowners Are as Burdened by Housing Costs as Renters," *Urban Wire* (blog), June 14, 2017; G. Thomas Kingsley, "Trends in Housing Problems and Federal Housing Assistance," Urban Institute, October 26, 2017. For more about the Bay Area housing market, see Kathleen Pender, "One-Third Rule Not Always Feasible in Bay Area Rental Market," *San Francisco Chronicle,* March 10, 2014.

13. Pearl Braveman et al., "How Does Housing Affect Health?," Robert Wood Johnson Foundation, May 1, 2011, https://www.rwjf.org/en/library /research/2011/05/housing-and-health.html.

14. Kathryn Leifheit et al., "Eviction in the United States: Affected Populations, Housing and Neighborhood-Level Consequences, and Implications for Health," Society for Epidemiologic Research Meeting, 2018.

15. Matthew Desmond and Rachel Kimbro, "Eviction's Fallout: Housing, Hardship, and Health," *Social Forces* 94, no. 1 (2015): 295–324, doi: 10.1093/sf/sov044.

16. Sandra J. Newman and C. Scott Holupka, "Housing Affordability and Investments in Children," *Journal of Housing Economics* 24 (2014): 89–100; Fredrik Andersson et al., "Childhood Housing and Adult Earnings: A Between-Siblings Analysis of Housing Vouchers and Public Housing," National Bureau of Economic Research (October 2016), working paper 22721.

17. Daniel Engster and Helena O. Stensota, "Do Family Policy Regimes Matter for Children's Well-Being?," *Social Politics: International Studies in Gender, State and Society* 18, no. 1 (March 7, 2011): 82–124, doi: 10.1093 /sp/jxr006.

18. See Glenn Thrush, "Here Is a Guide to Biden's Three Big Spending Plans—Worth About $6 Trillion," *New York Times,* April 28, 2021.

19. For more about the positive impact of paid-family-leave policies, see Katherine Policelli and Alix Gould-Werth, "New Research Shows California Paid Family Leave Reduces Poverty," Washington Center for Equitable Growth, August 20, 2019; "Paid Leave Will Help Close the Gender Wage Gap," National Partnership for Women and Families, 2018; Jacob Klerman et al., "Family and Medical Leave in 2012: Technical Report," prepared for the U.S. Department of Labor, September 7, 2012.

About This Project

1. Since its founding in 1971, CSPI has advocated for clearer federal nutrition advice, food and menu labeling, improved school food, and less food and beverage marketing, specifically to children. It also has research arms, which inform aspects of its advocacy work.

2. For the report generated from this research, see Priya Fielding-Singh, Jessica Almy, and Margo Wootan, "Sugar Overload: Retail Checkout Promotes Obesity," Center for Science in the Public Interest, 2014.

3. In this book, I mainly refer to parents' income backgrounds. However, in the original research design, I used a composite measure to determine a family's socioeconomic status that combined parents' education and household income. High-socioeconomic families had at least one parent with a college education and a household income above 350 percent of the poverty line. In middle-socioeconomic families, both parents had at least a high-school education and a household income between 180 and 350 percent of the poverty line. Some of these families had parents with a college or associate's degree. In low-socioeconomic families, neither parent had more than a high-school degree, and the household income didn't exceed 180 percent of the poverty line. For reference, students in a family of four qualify for free lunches if their household income is $31,525 or less and reduced-price lunches if their household income is between $31,526 and $44,863. In this study, a family of four was classified as middle-socioeconomic if its household income was between $44,863

and $85,050. A family of four was classified as a high-socioeconomic family if its household income exceeded $85,050. Within each socioeconomic bracket, I interviewed roughly equal numbers of self-identified Black, Asian, Latinx, and white families. For more information about the sample, see Priya Fielding-Singh, "A Taste of Inequality: Food's Symbolic Value Across the Socioeconomic Spectrum," *Sociological Science* (August 2017).

4. While most families in my study with two parents were headed by different-sex couples, I also interviewed a handful of same-sex couples. However, given the small number of these families within my sample—and, accordingly, my uncertainty about to what degree these families' experiences were reflective of other same-sex couples' experiences—I made the decision not to include their stories in the book. For research on housework, foodwork included, among same-sex couples, see Abbie E. Goldberg, "'Doing' and 'Undoing' Gender: The Meaning and Division of Housework in Same-Sex Couples," *Journal of Family Theory and Review* 5, no. 2 (2013): 85–104.

5. I had every single interview I conducted transcribed verbatim. I had interviews that I conducted in Spanish transcribed in Spanish and then translated to English. I triangulated these transcription data with my field notes to reconstruct scenes for the book.

6. When I was ready to write this book, I read and reread every interview and field note several times. As I wrote, I prioritized my firsthand observations and secondhand information that had been confirmed by multiple family members. Once the book was written, I recontacted Nyah, Dana, Renata, and Julie and read them relevant portions of the book to check factual details. I used the qualitative-data-analysis software Dedoose for all analyses of interviews and field notes for peer-reviewed academic publications whose arguments and findings provided a basis for this book. In writing the actual book itself, I did not use qualitative-data software.

Index

About the Author

Priya Fielding-Singh is an assistant professor in the Department of Family and Consumer Studies at the University of Utah, where she researches, teaches, and writes about families, health, and inequality in America. She earned her PhD in sociology from Stanford University and completed her postdoctoral training as a National Institutes of Health Fellow in Cardiovascular Disease Prevention at the Stanford University School of Medicine. Her research and writing examine issues of social, economic, and racial justice, with a focus on food and nutrition equity.